the METABOLIC STORM

SECOND EDITION

The science of
your metabolism and
why it's making you FAT
and possibly INFERTILE

P.S. It's not your fault

Emily Cooper, M.D.

Published 2013
ISBN: 978-0-9896902-0-1
Library of Congress Control Number: 2013913572

For information, address:
Seattle Performance Medicine, PLLC
2320 W. Commodore Way, Suite 100
Seattle, WA 98199

To my grandmother, Ella K. Cooper, M.D.,
who graduated from medical school in 1914 and
inspired me to practice preventive medicine.

And to my father, Edward K. Cooper, who still brings
laughter and joy to all of our lives.

And to my mother, Janice O. Cooper, close advisor, who
inspires us all to live life to the fullest.

Contents

Introduction

THIS IS NOT A DIET BOOK.

I won't tell you that cutting out bread, eating less, exercising more, juicing kale, or tracking "calories in, calories out" with the latest apps will solve a weight problem.

Why not?

Because of the thousands of patients I've treated over the past twenty-five years, only an alarming few have experienced long-term resolution of their weight problems as a result of dieting and exercising.

But don't worry—there's good news! In the pages to follow, I will share with you what I have learned in my many years of medical practice regarding weight and metabolism. Great scientific advances have been made in recent years that have helped to explain how hormones and metabolism regulate weight gain and loss. For the treatment of obesity, today's science brings great hope. This new edition brings more personal stories, scientific explanations and new research about weight regulation. I've also included a new chapter explaining how metabolism may affect your fertility.

BECOMING SHERLOCK HOLMES

I'm a Seattle-based physician, board certified in Family Medicine, Sports Medicine, and Obesity Medicine. As a medical student training in London, I was exposed to a *systems* approach to medicine, where diagnosis and treatment focus on the body as a whole rather than a fragmented system made up of individual parts. For example, I learned to examine a patient's abdomen as part of the *entire* gastrointestinal system, including the eyes, mouth, hands, and neck. In contrast, when U.S. medical students are asked to examine a patient's abdomen, their exam starts and ends with the abdomen.

While in London, I also learned to diagnose conditions by talking with patients and taking careful patient histories—not just identifying physical signs of disease, but exploring the underlying causes of disease. This approach takes time, patience, and the curiosity to explore the grey areas that exist between health and disease. It is like detective work. In the U.S., I've found that this kind of in-depth exploration is difficult to perform; our average seven-minute doctor-patient interaction leaves little time for deeper investigative work and exploration of those grey areas.

I began to learn about weight and metabolic issues in the 1980s, during my family medicine residency program. This was a period during which preventive medicine was the newest movement in medical care. Researchers were discovering that several health conditions were associated with increased body weight. They had just learned that type 2 diabetes was actually preventable, and that it was associated with insulin resistance and metabolic syndrome. Ultimately, researchers linked the causes of diabetes, cholesterol problems, high blood pressure, and overweight conditions together as one larger condition. They referred to it as *syndrome X* at the time; later, they began to call it *metabolic syndrome* or *dysmetabolic syndrome*.

I was very excited to learn about insulin resistance and metabolic syndrome, because if they were indeed reversible and preventable, we had found a new avenue for making a real difference in preventing weight problems, diabetes, heart attacks, and strokes. My interest in this area of medicine grew in the 1990s, when some of my patients were gaining weight in spite of their efforts to lose or maintain weight. Some of them appeared to be affected by all of the conditions that make up metabolic syndrome; some were affected by only a few of them. Other patients were very healthy, yet they still had problems controlling their weight. Many of my patients kept detailed records about what they ate, their exercise regimen, how much they slept, etc.—and in the majority of cases, this meticulously collected data didn't add up based on the conventional "calories in, calories out" theory. This caught my attention, and it became a puzzle that I am still investigating to this day.

DEAD ENDS

Twenty years ago, I thought that all I needed to do to help my overweight patients was to educate them on healthy eating and exercise. This was naïve of me. Granted, at the time (as in the present) this was the standard approach— but it was a short-term strategy at best. Some patients experienced no change in weight whatsoever; others experienced drastic drops of up to one hundred pounds. Regardless of how much weight was lost, however, it always came back. The more patients I treated, the clearer it became: this approach was not working. I was frustrated. It was discouraging to both my patients and me to find that even if we succeeded in the short term, the weight that was lost—and often even more than that—eventually returned.

USING AN OLYMPIC MINDSET

When the diet and exercise approach failed me, I decided to put my sports science experience to use. Sports science focuses on finding out what makes athletes perform, to help them reach goals like a personal best, breaking a world record, getting to the Olympics, winning a medal, or making a professional team. With this focus in mind, in 1999 I launched a more scientific approach to tackle my patients' weight issues: I began using high-tech equipment to measure their metabolisms instead of relying on standard predictive formulas based on height, weight, gender and age. Over the following months, I had my patients wear a mask that measured their breath to determine what their metabolic rate was before and after meals, how it was affected by one food versus another, and what it was before, during, and after exercise. I thought this method would allow me to fine-tune the "calories in, calories out" formula—that in matching my approach to each patient's specific test results I could be more accurate than the textbook calculations I had previously used. Based on this strategy, I drafted individual eating and exercise plans calculated to effect weight loss in each patient.

WEIGHT LOSS 2.0 FAILS

To my surprise and dismay, though I had perfected the "calories in, calories out" equation, tailoring it to my patients based on their individual metabolic tests, the new results were no better than the previous results. Patients who did respond to my treatment plan only kept the weight off temporarily. Patients could eat all the "right" foods and exercise "correctly" and still have trouble losing their excess weight, maintaining the weight they lost, or keeping their weight from increasing. In spite of all the science and technology I had at my fingertips, I could not get my patients' bodies to respond in any meaningful way.

THE UNLIKELY ANOREXIA CONNECTION

As I analyzed my patients' metabolisms and blood work, I noticed striking similarities to those of my patients with anorexia. I realized that patients with obesity and patients with anorexia, including those who were severely underweight, had far more in common metabolically than most people would ever suspect. Their blood work showed that both their bodies thought they were starving. How could someone's overweight body feel it was as starving as someone's underweight body? I first suspected that my overweight patients' low-calorie and low-carb dieting history had caused this confusion in their body—but over time I learned that while that contributed to their problems, it was more complicated than that.

BETTER SCIENCE

I thought I was being scientific in measuring each patient's metabolism to find the right formula for weight loss, but it turned out I was not being scientific enough! As I looked at all the data, I realized that the "calories in, calories out" solution to long-term weight management is ancient history (it was first popularized between 1910 and 1930) and terribly inadequate. It was with great relief that my search led me to a treasure trove that explained *what really drives weight problems.* I began to challenge antiquated assumptions and embrace a purely scientific perspective, not based on speculation, but based on scientific observation, not what scientists *presumed* should apply but what they *proved* applied in real life. This perspective would finally allow me to help my patients begin to navigate their weight problems in an informed and more effective way.

Today, the majority of patients I treat in my clinical practice have experienced significant improvements in their health, metabolism, and weight by applying a scientific approach rather than by dieting and engaging in extreme exercise.

THERE'S HOPE

In this book, I will explain to you why diet and exercise are not a cure for weight problems, and I will explain the complex science of overweight and obesity in a way that's easy to understand. You'll learn why obesity is actually caused by a medical condition—not a behavioral problem, as many would have you believe—and how weight and health are not the same thing.

Next, I'll introduce you to hormones and how they communicate with the brain to control your body weight. We'll delve into common problems that affect the metabolism, appetite, and weight, and I'll explain how these problems add up to what I call the *Metabolic Storm,* where the information feedback loop between your body and brain that keeps weight in balance is thrown off and malfunctions. We'll also talk about typical hormonal imbalances that lead to weight problems and their symptoms. I'll explain the metabolism's influence in other areas like thyroid, cortisol and fertility. Along the way, I'll share stories and comments from patients who have faced these struggles and experienced the symptoms of metabolic dysfunction.[1]

In the following pages I will present scientific evidence that diets slow the metabolism down, creating an effect that I call *Diet Fog.* You will learn that weight regain after dieting is not the result of having stopped dieting, but rather a result of the fact that the diets stop working as Diet Fog sets in. We'll discuss how dieting can precipi-

---

1. All patients have given consent to publish their stories and comments. Their names have been changed to protect their privacy.

tate an acceleration of metabolic disturbance—so much so that it can sometimes cause an out-of-control imbalance in the metabolic system, what I call the Metabolic Storm. This Storm can escalate to a Category 5 hurricane, leading to rapid weight gain. We'll talk about the current state of belief in the medical community regarding weight problems and whether they constitute a disease. We'll talk about the current groundbreaking guidelines for healthcare providers and obstacles in the healthcare system that obstruct application of these new guidelines. And finally, I will introduce you to promising new treatments and approaches that can help calm the Metabolic Storm for the majority of people, making future obesity treatment better for everyone.

In understanding how the metabolism works, you'll come to realize why no matter what plan you choose, deprivation diets don't work long term for the vast majority of people. You don't fail at dieting; it's the diets that fail you. And today's science offers great hope. As one of my patients said so succinctly, "I always knew there was science. I always believed there was a physiological explanation."

Finally, all of us deserve to know that weight problems are not our fault.

CHAPTER 1

Fat Prejudice: The Last Acceptable Bias

OVER THE PAST ONE HUNDRED years, scientists have discovered numerous hormones that are involved in weight regulation. We now have at our fingertips an enormous body of published scientific research describing the millions of chemical reactions that take place in the body and are collectively responsible for controlling body weight, metabolism, and appetite.

In spite of all this scientific knowledge, there is no current consensus among physicians or insurers in the U.S. about whether overweight and obesity even *are* a medical problem. Like the general public, many healthcare providers believe weight issues are caused by behavioral or emotional problems, a theory that was first heavily promoted in the 1950s.

Recently, however, even the conservative American Medical Association (AMA) announced that it voted to classify obesity as a disease. In fact, the AMA agreed with the American Heart Association (AHA) that obesity is a "multi-metabolic hormonal disease state." In doing so, the AMA joins The American Society for Metabolic and Bariatric Surgery (ASMBS), The Obesity Society (TOS), The American Society of Bariatric Physicians (ASBP), and the American Association of Clinical Endocrinologists (AACE) in regarding obesity as a disease.

This viewpoint is still far from universal among medical professionals and the general public, but regardless of their position on whether weight difficulties are a medical or a behavioral/emotional problem, everyone agrees on one thing: we are facing an obesity epidemic in the U.S. today.

Consider this: if overweight and obesity were caused by behavioral or emotional problems it would mean that the 30 percent of the U.S. population who are in the normal weight range are the only people in the country who are in control of their behavior. This isn't logical, of course. Or true.

There is another explanation: biological factors, not behavioral flaws, are the root cause of weight problems.

Prominent organizations recognize OBESITY as a DISEASE.

☑ World Health Organization (1948)
☑ National Institutes of Health (1998)
☑ Centers for Disease Control (1998)
☑ Social Security Administration (1999)
☑ The Centers for Medicare and
   Medicaid Services (2004)
☑ The Endocrine Society (2005)
☑ The Obesity Society (2008)
☑ American Association of Clinical
   Endocrinologists (2012)*
☑ American Medical Association (2013)*
☑ Food and Drug Administration
☑ National Heart, Lung and Blood Institute
☑ American Heart Association*

*refer to obesity as a "multimetabolic
and hormonal disease state"

Yet a minority of medical professionals and the public view obesity as a medical condition.

Medical Professionals
24%

General Public
15%

©2015 Emily Cooper, M.D.

Since the early 1900s, but especially in the last two decades, researchers have made incredible discoveries related to the intricacies of weight and metabolism regulation. Admittedly, the science of metabolism and weight
regulation is very complex; as a student of the topic, I can
attest to that. However, it's absolutely worth taking the
time to learn about the basics, especially if you or your
loved ones belong to the nearly 70 percent of people in
the U.S. who are overweight or obese.

BMI: FULL OF FLAWS

Overweight and obesity are commonly measured by BMI
(Body Mass Index). BMI, created in the 1800s by a stat-
istician, is a mathematical formula that determines the
ratio of a person's height to weight. But the formula ap-
plies the same way to everyone—whether you are male,
female, young, old, athletic, sedentary, or have a large
or small bone frame—and, in many cases, this one-size-
fits-all method of measuring what constitutes a normal
weight is an inaccurate indication of health and body fat.
Muscular men and large-boned women invariably fall
into the "overweight" or "obese" BMI categories, even
when they do not have excess body fat.

There are other ways to define obesity, such as by measuring the amount of body fat on an individual or by analyz-

ing the *location* of their body fat—for example, focusing on visceral fat (around organs). These measurements are much more accurate than the often misleading BMI formula.

BEING OVERWEIGHT IS NO PICNIC

Many of my overweight patients report a variety of symptoms, including, in some cases, preoccupation with food, feeling hungry all the time, not feeling satisfied after eating, fatigue, tight muscles and body aches.

Sometimes the only symptoms are discomfort related to the excess body fat itself. Jane, for example, who had struggled with obesity since her twenties, was told by doctors that other than her weight problem, she was in good health. But she was at her wit's end when she came to see me. A large amount of fat hung beneath her arms, making them feel so heavy that she was having trouble lifting them. "I feel like I have dumbbells attached to my arms!" she lamented. "It's miserable!"

Activities that others take for granted require a lot more physical work for people who carry extra weight. Daniel, who started dieting as a young boy, is now an amazing cyclist. When I tested his fitness, he was able to push as much power as competitive elite cyclists. His fitness level was right up there with those who finish toward the front of the pack at cycling races. But, because Daniel carries

The woman on the left has a BMI of 38, putting her in the obese category. In spite of her excess weight, her measured fitness level falls in the "very fit" category. The fitness level of the woman on the right, who is in the normal-weight category, falls in the "unfit" category.

©2015 Emily Cooper, M.D.

an extra one hundred pounds, a large part of his energy is dedicated to moving his body against gravity. So, in spite of the fact that he's more fit than most of his competitors, he finishes in the back of the pack in every event. No one who watched him compete would ever realize he's actually stronger than most of the group. This is why fitness cannot be accurately judged by BMI or by who finishes first.

When I told Cheryl her weight problem was the result of a medical problem, she said, "I can't tell you how often I've heard people say that my weight issues just boil down to how weak I am. I have to show I'm extra 'whatever' to make up for being fat. I've always had to organize my personality around proving myself." So many in our society see being thin as successful and heavy as a failure. Cheryl's story is so common and one I hear time after time: "I'm successful in every other area of my life, yet I just can't master this."

WEIGHT IS NOT THE PROBLEM, IT'S A SYMPTOM

Tom weighs more than 450 pounds. When he came to see me he was looking for help getting his weight down. Everyone was worried that he was going to have a stroke or a heart attack any minute. When I tested Tom, however, not only was his blood pressure in the optimal part of the normal range, but his cholesterol levels were, too.

Some people with high body weight do develop chronic diseases, such as diabetes, hypertension, heart disease, kidney failure, and some cancers. We often hear that carrying excess weight increases the risk of developing these and

Who do you think has pre-diabetes?

John

Sophia

©2015 Emily Cooper, M.D.

other diseases. But the science of obesity challenges that theory by pointing out that excess weight, high blood pressure, high blood sugar, and high cholesterol or triglycerides are frequently identified as symptoms of an underlying problem with a common root cause. Weight, therefore, is a symptom of an underlying problem, but not necessarily the root cause of many associated health concerns. In fact, researchers have found that 51 percent of overweight individuals and 32 percent of patients with obesity are healthy in terms of blood pressure, cholesterol, and blood glucose levels.[1]

1. R.P. Wildman, P. Muntner, K. Reynolds, et al., "The Obese Without Cardiometabolic Risk Factor Clustering and the Normal Weight With Cardiometabolic Risk Factor Clustering: Prevalence and Correlates of 2 Phenotypes Among the U.S. Population (NHANES 1999-2004)," Archives of Internal Medicine (August 11, 2008), 168(15), doi: 10.1001/archinte.168.15.1617: 1617-1624.

Sean weighs 165 pounds. When he came to see me, he was confused about why, in spite of years of experience as a rock climber and mountaineer, he couldn't improve his fitness. From the outside, one would judge Sean to be the picture of health. When I tested him, however, I found that his blood pressure was elevated, his heart arteries were filled with plaque, and he had pre-diabetes. We often assume that maintaining a normal weight is a sign of health, but in reality scientists have found that 24 percent of normal-weight people have chronic diseases that are often attributed only to people who are obese.

Children can also be affected by adult diseases, such as high cholesterol, high blood pressure and diabetes. John's mother was concerned because although he was only 15 and very athletic, John always seemed tired both on the field and at home. Since prediabetes and obesity run in her family, his mother thought it was important to have him screened for a possible medical condition. Sophia, now 15, had similar family risks of diabetes and obesity and had been seeing me since she was nine years old. From their appearances, most people assume that Sophia isn't as healthy as John, but to everyone's surprise, John was the one affected by prediabetes and elevated blood pressure, LDL particles and triglyceride levels (metabolic syndrome), while Sophia had normal levels. John and Sophia share their stories to illustrate that you can't tell how healthy a person is from the outside. It's what's inside that's most important. Everyone at risk should be screened regardless of their body weight, and, ideally, children should be screened starting at age ten if there is family history of diabetes (including gestational diabetes), high cholesterol, high blood pressure, or obesity, or if they are having symptoms. Metabolic problems in children often peak by age fourteen during the height of the growth spurt. If insulin resistance, pre-diabetes, type 2 diabetes, hypoglycemia, or metabolic syndrome are not detected early when many medical conditions are preventable, then problems can become long term and more difficult to reverse later in life. Fortunately, since John was screened early, after a year of medical treatment his blood sugar, LDL particles, blood pressure, and triglycerides became normal, and his energy levels improved. He's still working on eating all food groups regularly, fueling his exercise, getting plenty of sleep, and taking any medications or supplements prescribed. We will continue to follow his progress to make sure his metabolic system stays as healthy as possible as he completes his development.

I will explain in the coming chapters how excess weight is a symptom of a metabolism that isn't functioning normally, and how the underlying metabolic malfunctions that cause weight gain can sometimes trigger other medical conditions and diseases—such as high blood pressure, cholesterol problems, and diabetes and even infertility!

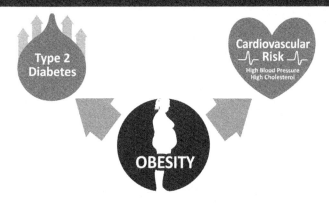

Obesity as root cause of cardiovascular risk and type 2 diabetes is a common misperception.

Type 2 Diabetes

Cardiovascular Risk
High Blood Pressure
High Cholesterol

OBESITY

Metabolic dysfunction is actually the root cause and excess weight is a symptom.

Type 2 Diabetes

Obesity

Cardiovascular Risk
High Blood Pressure
High Cholesterol

METABOLIC DYSFUNCTION

A weight problem is merely a visible sign of underlying metabolic disease—not the cause of poor health.

THE DIABESITY EPIDEMIC

Everyone knows that we are faced with a global obesity epidemic today, and the U.S. is in the top tier of countries affected. According to the Centers for Disease Control and Prevention (CDC), just under 70 percent of U.S. adults[2] were either in the overweight or obese weight ranges in 2010. They also found that more than one-third of American children and adolescents were in the overweight range and almost 20 percent were in the obese weight range.[3] This means that, according to the most recent data available, only about 30 percent of American adults and less than half of children are a normal weight. In addition to obesity trends climbing, experts project that by the year 2020 about 60 percent of the U.S. adult population will have either pre-diabetes or diabetes.[4] This combined epidemic of diabetes and obesity is often referred to as the

2. "Obesity and Overweight," *Faststats*, http://www.cdc.gov/nchs/fastats/overwt.htm.

3. "Childhood Obesity Facts," *Centers for Disease Control and Prevention*, http://www.cdc.gov/healthyyouth/obesity/facts.htm

4. M.D. Huffman, S. Capewell, H. Ning, et al., "Cardiovascular health behavior and health factor changes (1988-2008) and projections to 2020: Results from the National Health and Nutrition Examination Surveys," *AHA Circulation*, (May 2012), 125(21): 2595-2602.

Diabesity Epidemic. The term "diabesity" has been used in medical and scientific publications for decades as a way to link these two metabolic conditions which are frequently seen together.

Keith, a fourth-year medical student who rotated through my office, enjoyed working with our patients who were trying to get to the bottom of their weight-loss resistance. He spent much of his time at my practice learning about metabolism and how to diagnose common problems like metabolic syndrome, pre-diabetes, hypoglycemia (low blood sugar reactions) and insulin resistance.

Just as Keith was getting ready to move on to his residency program at a major university, he worried, "I won't be allowed to run these tests on my patients, will I?" Since obesity is not universally considered a treatable disease, the medical establishment and insurance companies theoretically have no justification for running tests to diagnose the underlying causes of obesity. As opposed to proactive, preventive medicine, where diagnosis and treatment are applied before a condition develops, the current medical philosophy in the U.S. is based on reactive treatment and short-term cost containment. The past couple of years has seen a little resurgence in the idea of preventive care but reimbursement for treatments with potential to effectively reverse obesity and pre-diabetes is unfortunately not considered necessary by many plans.

It is not until metabolic syndrome progresses to diabetes and cardiovascular disease that diagnosis and some of the most effective forms of treatment are covered consistently by insurance. I'm not an insurance expert but that doesn't strike me as a smart strategy for a country overloaded with these conditions. Most insurance plans in our country contain a clause about non-coverage for "weight related treatment." For example, a patient with insulin resistance and pre-diabetes, Carmen, told me recently that her previous doctor said a behavioral program was her only recourse for weight loss—there was nothing else he could do for her until she developed diabetes.

Many preventive tests are considered unnecessary because of our medical system's myopic focus on short-term cost containment in spite of a long-term burden on the system for everyone. When I was asked to evaluate Keith after his rotation, one of the top criteria for rating his expertise and performance was listed as his ability to demonstrate being "conscious of cost containment." According to the evaluation's rating scale of one to five, Keith could only receive a top score of five if he showed expertise in saving money in the short term.

Not only was Keith judged by more than his medical skills during his training, he was not taught about obesity as a disease in medical school. He told me that there was barely a mention of insulin resistance in his medical school textbooks and that he found only one paragraph about pre-diabetes in them as well. I checked for myself and found that the typical textbook used in medical school, "Current Medical Diagnosis & Treatment," is more than 1,700 pages long but dedicates only nine pages to diabetes and six pages to obesity. What's worse, one of the primary texts used in residency after medical school for doctors-in-training, "Harrison's Principles of Internal Medicine"—more than 3,500 pages long—devotes only 35 pages to diabetes and 14 pages to obesity, but includes 20 pages on bioterrorism and clinical medicine. Believe me, I want everyone to be safe. It's important. But should that subject really be given more attention than something that affects up to 70 percent of the U.S. population? In my twenty-five-year career, I've never witnessed a case of bioterrorism—but every year I see several hundreds of patients who are affected by pre-diabetes, diabetes, or obesity.

Health experts predict that the Diabesity Epidemic will affect 60 percent of adults in the U.S. within the next five to ten years, yet the doctors who will care for these affected people in the near future are not receiving adequate training to diagnose and treat obesity as a disease, as the "multi-metabolic hormonal disease state" that it's referred to by the AMA and AHA. In the long run, our lack of attention to this problem, especially in medical schools and residency training programs, will serve only to contribute to the epidemic's growth and mismanagement.

WHO'S HEALTHIER?

In addition to the myth that diets solve weight problems long term, "weight" and "health" have long been conflated and confused by popular culture. The truth is, many people of high body weight are healthy, and many are fit. The public perception is usually that weight and health are one and the same—that if you are thin you are healthier and more fit than someone who is overweight. However, as counterintuitive as it may seem, science actually suggests that once we reach a certain age we are healthier when we are at the top of the normal weight range or in the overweight range than we are when we're in the lower part of the normal range or in the underweight range.[5] Statistics show that normal-weight people do live longer than those who are in the underweight and extremely obese range. But you may be surprised to learn who lives longest of all: people in the overweight range![6]

WEIGHT AS A STIGMA

Despite all the groundbreaking scientific discoveries that have been made over the past two to three decades regarding the metabolic basis of obesity, research shows that weight discrimination is still very prevalent today, and

5. V. Hughes, "The big fat truth," *Nature,* May 2013.

6. Kaiser Permanente Center for Health Research, Underweight and Extremely Obese Die Earlier than People of Normal Weight, Study Finds, at http://www. kpchr.org/research/public/News.aspx?NewsID=35 (June 23, 2009).

that many people erroneously believe weight stigma is justified and can actually motivate people to lose weight.[7]

"I experienced unbelievable harassment at work from co-workers, to the point where I was uncomfortable eating around anybody," said one of my patients, who is a highly skilled nurse. "They would say, 'Fat people are lazy,' that we have no willpower. They would sit there and be talking about overweight people as though I were not even there. Ironically, I'm a very hard worker and can stick to something until it's done. I get a lot done on my to-do list, which takes a lot of willpower, right?"

I can't tell you how many patients have sat in my office in tears over offensive comments from a family member, friend, teacher, coach, co-worker, or, yes, healthcare provider who was trying to be "helpful."

"Fat equates to being lazy and undisciplined; I know that's what people think," Kate, whom you will learn more about in the following chapters, said. "It hurts me because I know I'm not undisciplined. I know that I'm strong mentally and I have strong discipline. It feels like my body has betrayed me. Everything I put in my mouth turns straight to fat. But no one wants to listen to me, so I don't even try."

Although she told her doctor that she was training for an

7. R.M. Puhl, C.A. Heuer, "Obesity Stigma: Important Considerations for Public Health," *American Journal of Public Health* (June 2010), Vol. 100, No. 6: 1019.

Ironman and still gaining weight, Kate said, "My doctor said, 'Honestly, I think that sometimes you just gotta buck up!'"

One of my patients, Amanda, told me about a terrible experience she had with an orthopedic surgeon recently. She had been trying hard to lose weight, participating in an intensive, boot camp-style diet and exercise program— and she suffered a hip injury in the course of the program. When she saw the orthopedist, he told her that she needed surgery but wasn't a candidate because she was "too big for the instruments."

Amanda, of course, was shocked.

"If you want surgery," the orthopedist then proceeded to say, "you need to lose weight. It's just calories in, calories out. It's a basic formula." To add insult to injury, the office walls were covered with photographs of the lean, fit orthopedist participating in triathlons. Amanda said it felt as if the photographs combined with the doctor's words were saying, "I'm better than you."

Researchers have reported that fat prejudice is rampant among healthcare professionals. "Basically, my past medical providers said, 'You can't possibly be eating that much and exercising that much and not losing any weight; it's not physically possible,'" recalled one of my patients. "Put down the fork," another person's doctor urged. What is said to children is possibly the most concerning and damaging: "You really have to stop eating the cookies," or

"You should lay off the computer games"—even when the child is not engaging in any of these behaviors.

Studies show that many nurses describe patients with obesity in negative terms and report that they tend to spend less time with someone who has obesity than they do with a person in what's considered a normal-weight patient range. In a study led by a Yale University psychologist, 35 to 48 percent of nurses said they feel "uncomfortable caring for obese people," and 31 to 42 percent said they'd "rather not care for them at all."[8]

Even obesity specialists demonstrate bias. The Yale study found that the stigma against people with weight problems is so strong that many people who study and treat obesity—people who understand that obesity is caused by a combination of genetic and environmental factors—believe that overweight people are lazy, stupid, and worthless. No wonder many people with weight problems avoid going to the doctor.

"If I have a cold, somehow it's due to my weight," one of my patients once told me. "If I have a sports-induced back sprain, it's most certainly thought to be due to my weight. No matter what my health issue, my doctors tend to blame my weight."

Many of my patients have reported that their experi-

---

8. M.B. Schwartz, et al. "Weight Bias among Health Professionals Specializing in Obesity," Obesity Research (September 2003), Vol. 11, No. 9.

ences with healthcare providers have frequently been frustrating and disheartening. And despite the vast body of science that suggests otherwise, excess weight is still usually not viewed as a medical problem but rather as a behavioral or emotional one, which means that patients are often left dealing with their health problems on their own.

BREAKING THE SPELL

The science of metabolism is very complicated, and it's up against a tremendous amount of widely dispersed misinformation. In the following chapters, you may read things that seem contrary to what you've heard before and different from theories and ideas in mainstream culture. Once you understand the science behind what is really going on inside your brain and body, I'm sure you will realize that excess body weight, infertility, and diabetes are not your fault.

CHAPTER 2

The Diet Myth

ALTHOUGH MOST PEOPLE—and even mainstream medicine—believe dieting is the only answer to weight loss, science demonstrates that there are more promising ways to deal with obesity. Dieting is not the only answer— in fact, it's not the answer at all. Diets may bring short-term success, but in the long run they nearly always fail. Just ask anyone who has been on a diet.

For many, dieting starts at a very young age. Many of my adult patients describe a childhood of locked cabinets and refrigerators, food hidden from sight, endless visits to the doctor or weight-loss clinics, even counting calories before they were fifteen years old. For others, however, it begins later in life—after a gradual or sudden weight gain.

I'd like to share my patient Kate's story with you. Like many of my patients, she was labeled "chubby" when she was a young girl, and she dieted for much of her life, beginning at age eleven. In spite of trying one diet after another, year after year, Kate could never get to her goal weight. Instead, she gained and lost the same five to fifteen pounds over and over again. "Diets never really worked for me," Kate recalled. This went on through her twenties and thirties until she finally gave up on dieting—at least for a while.

IT ALL COMES OFF

This changed when Kate, by now significantly over-weight, became fed up with her situation and decided to give her all to a program at her fitness club. Throughout the fifteen-month program, she meticulously adhered to a low-calorie diet and diligently kept up regular aerobic exercise. Through her persistent efforts, she lost eighty-five pounds and landed in a normal weight range. She was ecstatic. "I thought I had found the magic key to my weight problem," she said.

ATHLETE AT THE STARTING LINE

Kate maintained her new, lower weight for about two years, remaining careful about her dietary choices and portion sizes and exercising regularly. She had never been athletic before, but she realized that after two years of consistently working out she was fit and strong, and she enjoyed every aspect of exercise and fitness. "I wanted to run marathons," Kate said, "but my trainer suggested triathlons to protect my knees. Little did he know I would eventually participate in Ironman competitions, which include not only the marathons that I really wanted to run, but a 2.4-mile swim and a 112-mile bike ride *on top of* the marathon (26.2 miles), all in a continuous, one-day event!"

Like most Ironman athletes, as Kate ramped up her training she began to do fifteen to twenty hours of exercise per week, including workouts in all three sports: swimming, biking, and running. Many days included "brick" workouts, which are bike rides followed back-to-back by a run or a swim, followed immediately by a bike ride. Some days were double workout days: one in the morning and another in the afternoon.

TANKING UP? OR RUNNING ON FUMES?

Kate's Ironman workouts were meant to improve her endurance fitness. They burned about 500 calories per

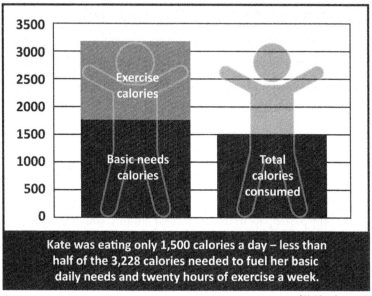

Kate was eating only 1,500 calories a day – less than half of the 3,228 calories needed to fuel her basic daily needs and twenty hours of exercise a week.

hour—which, since she was working out so much, translated to up to 10,000 calories per week. Someone her size usually needs around 1,800 calories a day just for day-to-day activities like dressing, showering, and going to work.

When it came to her training nutrition plan, Kate used the same basic strategy that had helped her lose eighty-five pounds: portion control, low-carb intake (though she allowed herself a little more carbs than before), low fat intake, and high protein intake. She continued to count calories meticulously. She increased her daily calorie intake to support her exercise—but only by 300 calories—from 1,200 to 1,500 calories.

If we do the math, Kate was eating only half of the calories per day that she needed to support her body size and workout schedule. She didn't realize that this new regimen actually represented a more extreme diet than she had ever been on before.

WHERE DID THE MAGIC GO?

Although this will be unfathomable to most people, Kate regained more than three quarters of the weight she had lost (sixty-five pounds) while training nearly twenty hours per week and consuming only 1,500 calories per day. She was devastated.

"At first I thought it was muscle, but more and more pounds kept coming on, and I got slower and slower," lamented Kate, who was participating in at least twelve triathlons each year at the time as part of her training.

"I kept trying to drop the weight, but it wasn't coming off, and worse, it was increasing steadily—even when I used the same methods I'd used to lose the original eighty-five pounds! I felt like I was stuck between a rock and a hard place. I asked myself, 'Where do I go from here? I can't eat less and I can't exercise more. So what do I do?'"

Kate, left, after losing 85 lbs and right, shortly after,
while ramping up her training for Ironman,
gaining back almost all of the weight she lost.

©2015 Emily Cooper, M.D.

WAKING THE SLEEPING TIGER

By the time Kate came to my office, she was completely frustrated and confused about what was going on.

"How did this happen?" she sobbed.

Like many patients struggling with their weight, we soon discovered that Kate had an undiagnosed medical problem that had caused her weight struggles since childhood—and it was a problem that diet and exercise could not cure. When she exercised so much while consuming a limited diet, Kate's condition caused her body to perceive her well-meaning tactics as deprivation, and this activated a powerful weight-defense system that made her body store all her fuel as fat for protection.

Like most people, Kate did not know that the body could carry so much extra fat and still feel deprived. When she found out that this was what was happening, she was stunned. "It just doesn't seem possible that you can diet and exercise your way to *more* weight. You are doing everything that people say will work, and it doesn't!"

THE DEEPER TRUTH

Everywhere we turn we hear, "Eat less and exercise more if you want to lose weight." People with higher body weight get this advice from well-meaning friends, co-workers, family members, athletic trainers, and healthcare providers. However, at least sixty years of scientific research has consistently shown that while diets do cause short-term weight loss, they don't produce significant or permanent long-term results in most overweight and obese people. And although every textbook on obesity clearly states this fact, very few people are aware of it. If diet and exercise didn't work for Kate, who was training nearly twenty hours per week and competing in Ironman events, what hope is there for everyone else? What better way to illustrate what science has been telling us for decades than with her story?

DIET SPORT

Dieting is a popular activity in the U.S., even among people of normal body weight. So many people—young and old, male and female, athletic and sedentary—are dieting. It's practically a hobby or a sport at this point. I always ask my patients who've never had a weight problem *why* they are dieting. The response is usually, "My friend was doing it, so I thought I'd try too," or, "Several of my co-workers recommended it." In our society, thinner is promoted as being better. No matter what we weigh, we think we should weigh less.

NO HARM DONE, RIGHT? WRONG.

Scientific evidence proving that dieting rarely solves weight problems in the long term is not new, but there's something else interesting about dieting: over the past sixty years, scientists have found that rather than helping with weight loss, diets can actually promote fu-

Deprivation diets slow metabolism by up to 36% within 6 months.

6 weeks after diet — 22% SLOWER

6 months after diet — 36% SLOWER

©2015 Emily Cooper, M.D.

ture weight *gain* because of their impact on metabolism. Almost all of my patients have experienced this devastating side effect of dieting, but until they came to see me, many of them had never before realized that the diet itself—which they viewed as successful in the short term— was what provoked their eventual weight gain.

Consider this common scenario: A sixteen-year-old girl of normal body weight goes on her first crash diet wanting to lose ten pounds to fit into a smaller sized junior prom dress. She successfully loses the weight in time for the prom, but afterwards begins to slowly regain the lost weight—and a then a little bit more. At seventeen, she

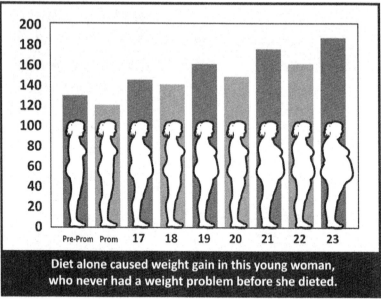

Diet alone caused weight gain in this young woman, who never had a weight problem before she dieted.

©2015 Emily Cooper, M.D.

goes on another diet and loses weight again, only to gradually regain the lost weight, plus even more. At twenty-five, the young woman, who never had a weight problem before her first diet, now weighs almost 200 pounds.

Scientists have found that dieting, especially for a child or adolescent, is associated with a higher rate of obesity in adulthood than it is for non-dieters. When normal-weight people repeatedly diet, sooner or later they are likely to trigger a metabolic problem, particularly if they are genetically inclined to have one. More often than not, they eventually find themselves seriously overweight and boxed into a corner because their diets stop working, even in the short term.

THE CALM BEFORE THE STORM

Most of my patients whose weight was elevated *before* their first diet have an underlying problem that hijacks the complex system that controls their metabolism. This chaotic disruption, which affects metabolism, weight, and appetite, is what I call the *Metabolic Storm.*

Dieting initially leads to a temporary shift in metabolism, which makes it seem at first like things are going very well. The appetite is calmer, weight is coming off, and energy levels are improving. As Kate said, it feels like you've found the "magic key" to your weight problems. But when a person has underlying metabolic problems, the body often doesn't accurately perceive the excess weight or the food supply signals properly, and due to the diet, it eventually begins to panic, perceiving starvation and storing fat for protection.

FOG SETS IN

Even when a diet gets off to a good start, before long the brain detects deprivation, and it interprets it as starvation. Even in overweight patients, the brain "sees" only the current deprivation triggered by dieting—it is blind to the excess weight, so it tells the body to store fat for protection.

This is the turning point—the moment in which the body stops letting go of excess weight. This deprivation detection causes weight-loss reversal. Scientists call this "biological adaptation" or "diet-induced weight defense." Once deprivation is detected, the body's weight-defense system activates. Lab reports can actually show this effect in what I refer to as *Diet Fog*, which is characterized by hormone and neurotransmitter changes that we will discuss later in the book. These most commonly include abnormally low leptin and fasting insulin levels and abnormally high ghrelin levels. These changes halt weight loss and trigger weight regain. Furthermore, Diet Fog is superimposed on the original problem that caused the excess weight in the first place, making it harder for a physician to see the big picture with routine lab testing. For example, a common metabolic problem, insulin resistance, is characterized by elevated fasting insulin levels, but since Diet Fog (biological adaptation to dieting) suppresses fasting insulin levels until they begin to normalize again, it's easy to miss insulin resistance on routine lab testing.

POURING GASOLINE ON THE FIRE

Over time, the metabolic irregularities caused by chronic dieting and the underlying medical issues that were originally impacting weight compound one another, catapulting people's weight higher than it was before they dieted. This uncontrollable weight rebound, which is often accompanied by constant hunger and reduced satiety, can cause individuals to revert to, and even surpass, their initial, pre-diet weight. As their weight increases again, after having lost weight in the short term, patients become extremely distressed, especially because they worked so hard to lose the weight in the first place. But often the more they try to lose weight, the more they gain. Their chronic Metabolic Storm has now become a raging, Category 5 hurricane. In fact, I have had patients who are gaining weight at a rate of 50% of their body weight per year, in spite of starving themselves.

Although diets may at first seem successful, scientists have found that by five years after starting a diet most people will have regained all the weight they lost—and a high percentage will weigh *more than* their pre-diet weight.[1]

THE TRUTH IS OUT THERE

Although you would never guess, based on the messages routinely promoted by the diet industry, the media, and even healthcare providers, the scientific research showing that diets are not effective long-term solutions is not only widely available in medical and scientific journals

1. T. Mann, A. J. Tomiyama, E. Westling, A. Lew, B. Samuels, J. Chatman, "Medicare's Search for Effective Obesity Treatments: Diets Are Not the Answer," *American Psychologist* (April 2007), Vol. 62, No. 3, doi: 10.1037/0003-066X.62.3.220: 220–233.

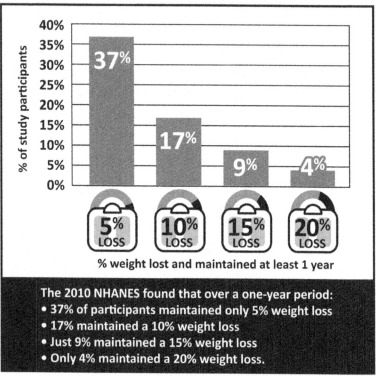

The 2010 NHANES found that over a one-year period:
• 37% of participants maintained only 5% weight loss
• 17% maintained a 10% weight loss
• Just 9% maintained a 15% weight loss
• Only 4% maintained a 20% weight loss.

©2015 Emily Cooper, M.D.

but also in every specialized advanced textbook written on the subject of obesity.

A study published in the *International Journal of Obesity*[2] in 2010, for example, examined the long-term weight-loss maintenance of 14,306 adults ages 20 to 84 who participated in the National Health and Nutrition Examination Survey (NHANES). NHANES is a series of interviews and

2. J. L. Kraschnewski, J. Boan, J. Esposito, et al., "Long-term weight loss maintenance in the United States," *International Journal of Obesity* (May 18, 2010), 34, doi:10.1038/ijo.2010.94: 1644–1654.

physical exams that the National Center for Health Statistics has conducted since 1971 to gauge the American public's health and nutritional status. The researchers discovered that among people who had been overweight or obese at some point in their life, 37 percent had maintained at least a five percent weight loss, 17 percent had maintained at least a 10 percent weight loss, 9 percent had maintained at least a 15 percent weight loss, and 4 percent reported keeping off at least a 20 percent weight loss for one year.

These results were reported as good news. The study concluded that one in six people maintained a weight loss of at least 10 percent in the long term (their definition of "long term" was at least one year), a higher percentage of long-term weight maintenance than researchers previously believed possible.

But let's take a closer look. The people who reported losing the greatest amount of weight were the least likely to keep the weight off. Even people who lost 5 percent of their weight had a relatively low success rate in weight-loss maintenance. Furthermore, there's a big catch: The researchers defined long-term weight loss as lasting one year or more. When someone has spent much of their life overweight or obese, a year is a very short time. Yes, most people who are overweight would love to lose even just 5 percent of their body weight, but they also want to keep that weight off—and most fail to do so.

Let's consider two hypothetical people: Mary, who at 5'4" weighs 200 pounds, and Walter, who at 5'10" weighs 300. Mary's BMI is 35, placing her in the "obese" category. Walter's BMI is 43, placing him in the "extremely obese" category.

Mary and Walter go on a diet to lose weight. The research shows that the odds are somewhat good (37 percent) that each will maintain a five percent weight loss for a year or more. This equates to ten pounds for Mary, bringing her to 190 pounds, and fifteen pounds for Walter, bringing him to 285 pounds.

The odds are less than half as good (17 percent) that they'll maintain the 10 percent weight loss that would bring Mary's weight to 180 (a 20-pound loss) and Walter's to 270 (a 30-pound loss). And if either wants to maintain a 15 percent weight loss, their chances of doing so drop almost in half again, to 9 percent—but if successful, Mary would weigh 170 pounds (a 30-pound loss) and Walter 255 pounds (a 45-pound loss).

At 4 percent, the odds are slim that either will maintain a 20 percent weight loss, which would bring Mary down to 160 pounds (a 40-pound loss) and Walter down to 240 pounds (a 60-pound loss).

It should be noted that if both Mary and Walter were able to lose 20 percent of their original body weight, Mary's BMI would still be in the overweight category and Walter's BMI would still be in the obese category. In spite of all their hard work and a slim chance of maintaining their weight loss, neither would have reached the normal weight category.

Another study published in the *International Journal of Obesity*[3] in 2005 found that whether study participants only dieted or dieted and exercised at the same time, by the one-year mark they had regained about 50 percent of their initial weight loss. The people who only dieted lost 22 pounds on average, while those who dieted and exercised lost an average of 29 pounds. Yet for all their hard work and great initial results, by the end of one year the people who only dieted regained 10 of their 22 pounds lost, and those who dieted and exercised regained 15 of their 29 pounds lost. And if they gained this much back before the end of the first year, what is to stop all the weight from coming back?

THE TRUTH BEHIND THE NUMBERS

In a study published in the journal *American Psychologist*[4] in 2007, researchers from UCLA set out to identify which obesity interventions should be funded under re-

3. C.C. Curioni, P.M. Lourenço, "Long-term weight loss after diet and exercise: a systematic review," *International Journal of Obesity* (May 31 2005), 29, doi:10.1038/sj.ijo.0803015: 1168–1174.

4. T. Mann, A.J. Tomiyama, E. Westling, et al., "Medicare's search for effective obesity treatments: diets are not the answer," *American Psychologist* (April 2007), 62(3): 220 233.

vised Medicare guidelines that cover only proven obesity treatments. They looked at fourteen studies that examined long-term (defined as being up to five years) results of calorie-restrictive diets. The UCLA researchers discovered that, conservatively, "from one third to two thirds of diet participants will weigh *more* four to five years after the diet ends than they did before the diet began."

"Many of the studies examined likely underestimate the extent to which dieting is counterproductive because of several methodological problems, all of which bias the studies toward showing successful weight-loss maintenance," the UCLA study authors wrote. In other words, the diets studied often left people worse off, not better off. And the way the studies were designed made their results indicate that people had more success in keeping their weight off than they actually had. The authors also noted that just because a study ended and the researchers stopped following up with participants, it didn't mean that the weight gain had stopped. They noted that even in studies "with the longest follow-up times (of four or five years post diet), the weight regain trajectories did not typically appear to level off, suggesting that if participants were followed for even longer, their weight would continue to increase."

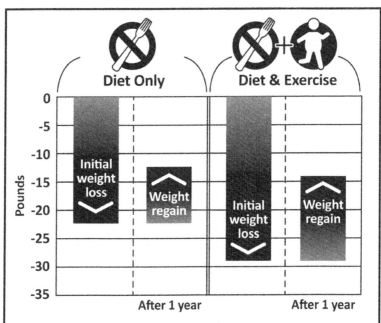

A study published in the International Journal of Obesity in 2005 found that regardless of whether study participants only dieted or dieted and exercised at the same time, by the one-year mark they still had regained about 50% of their initial weight loss.

HOW MANY DIETS HAVE YOU TRIED?

With decades of scientific research showing that dieting is a dead end for most people, you'd think that it would be out of style by now. But—understandably—people are looking for answers, and peer pressure to diet is very strong, even for normal-weight people. So for those who do suffer from weight problems, it's easy to imagine the immense pressure from family, co-workers, friends, and healthcare providers to dial up the dieting and exercise and keep "trying harder."

"I've been on thirty-two diets in my life, all prescribed by physicians," one of my patients told me. "I've been on a life-long diet and I'm at my all-time high body weight," is another common complaint. And as one patient recently lamented, "I started dieting when I was eight, yet at fifty I'm now heavier than ever!"

WHY DO WE DO THIS TO OURSELVES?

The massive "Handbook of Obesity: Clinical Applications, Third Edition" is one of the bibles of obesity medicine. In it, Robert F. Kushner, M.D., M.S., clinical director of Northwestern University medical school's Comprehensive Center on Obesity, and Louis J. Aronne, clinical professor of medicine and director of the Comprehensive Weight-Control Program at New York-Presbyterian Hospital/ Weill Cornell Medical Center, question why patients keep trying to lose weight even though their previous attempts haven't produced long-term results. They write:

> Given our current state of knowledge and the treatments currently available, the goal of obesity treatment should be the lowest weight the patient can comfortably maintain, which in the

average patient is about 5-10% loss of total body weight. Attaining ideal body weight or a loss of 20% of body weight is not possible for the vast majority of overweight and obese people.[5]

This means that at best, our hypothetical, 200-pound Mary would probably be able to lose only between ten and twenty pounds and keep it off, and 300-pound Walter could probably only maintain a fifteen- to thirty-pound weight loss.

Consider what University of Toronto psychologists Janet Polivy, PhD, and C. Peter Herman, PhD, both obesity researchers, write in a chapter of "Handbook of Obesity" titled *Weight Cycling as an Instance of False Hope:*[6]

People do tend to succeed in the early stages of weight loss attempts and most dieters have at least some early success to spur them on. When weight loss slows or stops, however, people tend to become vulnerable to elements that interfere with further weight loss. The weight loss attempt is judged to have failed. Over time, however, most people experience a renewed desire to lose

5. R.F. Kushner, L.J. Aronne, "Obesity and the Primary Care Physician," *Handbook of Obesity: Clinical Applications, Third Edition, ed.* George A. Bray and Charles Brouchard (New York, Informa, 2008), 125.
6. J. Polivy, C.P. Herman, "Weight Cycling as an Instance of False Hope," *Handbook of Obesity: Clinical Applications, Third Edition, ed.* George A. Bray and Charles Brouchard (New York: Informa, 2008), 105.

weight, and begin a new weight loss program or effort. This subsequent effort usually follows the same pattern.

That is to say, diets tend to work at first—at least somewhat. But over the long term, most people regain the weight and more, in spite of multiple dieting attempts.

YES, EVEN THE TEXTBOOKS ARE SAYING THIS

It is bad enough to experience the heartbreak and frustration of gaining lost weight back. But what most people don't realize is that science proves that not only does dieting stand virtually no chance of working, it often makes an existing weight problem worse. Polivy and Herman continue:

> *Weight cycling may have metabolic effects that make subsequent weight loss efforts more difficult and contribute to subsequent obesity. Given that weight cycling appears to increase the risk of overweight/obesity, however, it seems likely that weight cycling may contribute to these problems through its ultimately elevating effect on body weight. Weight cycling thus appears to*

entail at least some risk, if only from the ratch-
eting upward of weight that seems to result
from cycles of success and failure at weight loss.[7]

Translation: dieting impacts the metabolism in ways that increase the odds that people will eventually gain weight above and beyond their starting weight. As many of my patients might say, "diets make you fatter". Being well aware of this information, I'm never surprised when this happens but unfortunately, most patients and even some physicians are not prepared for the diet backlash that inevitably occurs. One of my new patients was horrified that although she had lost 50 pounds at a medical weight-loss center on a 'ketogenic diet' (extremely low carb), she had gained back 30 pounds and had a higher body fat percentage than she did when she started. She was shocked when I explained that she responded to the prescribed diet just like anyone else would have and exactly as textbooks predicted she would. She lost lots of weight initially, not just fat, but muscle and water weight as well. Like most people who follow very low carb diets, what she regained was almost all fat. So while her body weight landed at a lower level, the percentage of body fat was greater than when she started.

7. J. Polivy, C.P. Herman, "Weight Cycling as an Instance of False Hope," *Handbook of Obesity: Clinical Applications, Third Edition, ed.* George A. Bray and Charles Brouchard (New York: Informa, 2008), 113.

In a classic obesity medicine text, "Obesity Prevention and Treatment," George A. Bray, MD, chief of the division of clinical obesity and metabolism at Pennington Biomedical Research Center at Louisiana State University, describes similar limitations:

> *Results from most long-term clinical studies of treatment for overweight patients show a high prevalence of weight regain. In the Institute of Medicine report "weighing the options" for those who achieved weight loss, more than one-third of the weight typically was regained within one year and nearly all within five years.*[8]

Again, according to these authors it's unrealistic to expect to keep lost weight off with dieting. Whatever people lose, they're going to gain back by the end of Year Five.

It's worth noting that the report *Weighing the Options: Criteria for Evaluating Weight Management Approaches*[9] was published by a nonprofit, non-governmental health arm of the National Academy of Sciences (NAS), an organization that provides decision-makers

---

8. G.A. Bray, "Classification and Evaluation of the Overweight Patient," Handbook of Obesity: Clinical Applications, Third Edition, ed. George A. Bray and Charles Brouchard (New York: Informa, 2008), 23.

9. Committee to Develop Criteria for Evaluating the Outcomes of Approaches to Prevent and Treat Obesity, Institute of Medicine, *Weighing the Options: Criteria for Evaluating Weight Management Approaches, ed.* Paul R. Thomas (Washington, D.C.: National Academies Press, 1995).

and the public with what its website describes as "unbiased and authoritative advice." The study was published way back in 1995, when Windows was a cutting-edge innovation, most people were just beginning to use email, and no one had ever even heard of Instagram. Almost twenty years have passed since the study was published, and this scientific knowledge has been replicated countless times since then, yet somehow this well-established information has not broken through the massive dieting messaging in popular culture.

Of course, research like this is often buried in obscure medical publications with titles like *Clinical Obesity* and *Current Opinion in Endocrinology, Diabetes and Obesity*—not the typical publications you would download onto your Kindle, find on the newsstand, or read on the treadmill or in your doctor's waiting room.

SCIENCE NEEDS BETTER PUBLIC RELATIONS—WHAT'S THE HOLDUP?

It's not unusual for there to be a significant lag between when scientists make a discovery and when the medical establishment adopts the change or pharmaceutical companies invent medications that apply the new knowledge. And it takes even longer before the medications become available to the public. For example, it's not unusual for up to twenty years to pass between an important scientific discovery and the time it shows up in a medical school textbook. When it comes to metabolism discoveries, in many cases decades have passed before proven science has made its way into textbooks.

There are probably many reasons why the myth about diets' effectiveness has stuck around like gum on the bottom of a shoe. One valid rationale is that the actual science is extremely complicated. Understanding the metabolism requires a good amount of scientific knowledge and specialized study. As I mentioned in Chapter One, metabolism and weight problems are barely touched on during medical school, and once doctors are out in practice their time is limited, so many are likely to find it overwhelming to keep up with all the current research.

There are other challenges faced by the science of metabolism and obesity. In 1995, an Institute of Medicine study noted that the weight-loss industry was worth billions of dollars.[10] Today, the industry is worth some $60 billion.[11] An industry with this much capital behind it has the power to give antiquated ideas tremendous weight and dissuade the American public from believing the countering science. And the weight-loss industry isn't

10. Committee to Develop Criteria for Evaluating the Outcomes of Approaches to Prevent and Treat Obesity, Institute of Medicine, *Weighing the Options: Criteria for Evaluating Weight Management Approaches*, ed. Paul R. Thomas (Washington, D.C.: National Academies Press, 1995).

11. Brooke Axtel, "How to Be A Shameless Woman: Making Peace With Our Bodies, Ourselves," *Forbes*, September 26, 2012.

the only industry whose existence is predicated upon this erroneous, outdated information; the media, the fitness industry, the supplements industry, book publishing, and other industries have extended these ideas' longevity as well.

We should also keep in mind that people long for an overnight fix, a miracle diet that will solve their weight problem for good. Out of desperation, they may ignore what their past experiences prove, let alone what science proves—that their diets don't work long term, and that the weight eventually comes back in spite of all their efforts.

CHAPTER 3

Hormone Handbook: Beyond Estrogen and Testosterone

"I'VE ALWAYS DREAMED there was a problem with my metabolism that caused my body to hold on to fat," Sarah said, "but I didn't know there really WAS a problem!"

Counter to what we have all been told, weight problems really are commonly caused by metabolism problems. In this chapter, I will introduce many little-known but powerful hormones that play a major role in regulating weight, metabolism, and appetite.

A normally functioning metabolic feedback loop leads to high energy, calm appetite and stable body weight.

A dysfunctional metabolic feedback loop often leads to low energy, high appetite and excess body weight.

BRAIN IS BOSS

Our weight, metabolism, and appetite are controlled by a complex system. The brain and body communicate in a feedback loop where the brain is the CEO and the hormones produced in the body are the messengers. These hormonal messengers provide important information about our body weight and fuel supply by using what is called the *peripheral metabolic pathway* to get their signals to the brain. Within the brain, the *central metabolic pathway* interprets those incoming signals and sends its own output signals back to the body.

WE'VE COME A LONG WAY

Over the past twenty years in particular, many scientists have dedicated their entire career to studying these interrelated pathways. The science is complicated, but what scientists are clear about is the basic physiology of the system that regulates our metabolism, the areas where glitches can occur, the ways that we can potentially treat these glitches medically, and why diets don't work long-term. Treatments available now and those in development offer promising strategies for repairing problems along this critical pathway. New scientific research in the area of metabolism, overweight, and obesity is now progressing at such an explosive pace that it's impossible to keep up with it all. As a physician working with patients on these

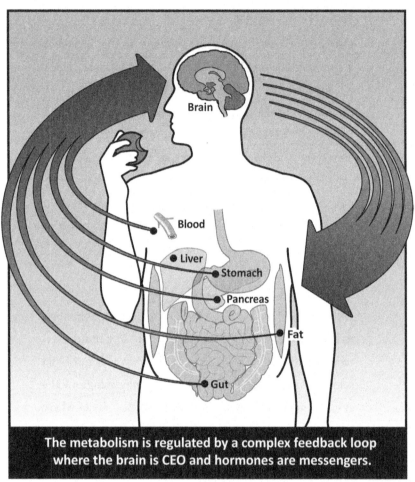

The metabolism is regulated by a complex feedback loop where the brain is CEO and hormones are messengers.

©2015 Emily Cooper, M.D.

problems, these fascinating new discoveries and promising inventions are already helping so many patients. I cannot wait to see what the next ten years bring.

MIXED SIGNALS

My biggest breakthrough came the moment I realized that similar metabolic issues can be caused by either *perceived* underweight and malnutrition (which, interestingly, occurs in most patients who are weight prone and weight-loss resistant) or *actual* underweight and malnutrition (found in patients who are underweight or with anorexia nervosa). These two types of people have a number of common blood test results, symptoms, and physical findings. For instance, hormone levels, body temperature, satiety, and fertility may be similarly affected in both groups, and female patients with obesity may even stop having regular menstrual periods, just as patients with anorexia stop menstruating.

I knew that science supported this finding. However, it wasn't until I finally measured and compared the labs of my overweight and underweight patients that I saw exactly how close the body's experience of perceived starvation is to actual starvation.

The people in the photos on the following page had similar blood levels of a neurotransmitter that signals starvation.

The metabolic feedback loop and its hormone messengers dictate the brain and body's perception of nourishment and weight. They adjust the metabolism, bodyweight, and apetite according to that perception– whether it's real or not. Faulty hormone levels or signals

The patient on the left has a BMI of about 12 due to anorexia. The patient on the right has a BMI of about 60 due to metabolic dysfunction. These two people have common blood test results, symptoms and physical findings indicating underweight status and malnutrition (real and perceived).

lead the brain and body to perceive that a person is underweight or undernourished, even if this is not true.

Susan could not understand why she couldn't lose any weight and why she actually gained weight when she lowered her food intake to only 800 calories per day. After looking at her lab work, I noted that her level of leptin, a hormone that informs the brain of the body's fat mass, was abnormally low.

"What do you mean?" Susan asked. "My brain thinks my weight is one hundred pounds lower than it really is? I would be really underweight if that were true!"

In this type of situation the metabolism reacts as though the individual is seriously underweight and malnourished, causing the body to desperately increase body weight and appetite, attempting to counter what it erroneously thinks is a life-threatening situation. This is why diets don't work: weight problems are often the body's way of trying to protect itself from a wrong perception of starvation. Diets only make that perception stronger over time. Once you understand more about how hormones of metabolism function, this will become clearer.

MEET YOUR HORMONES

Endocrine tissue manufactures and secretes *hormones* into the bloodstream and the nervous system. Hormones are chemical messengers, produced by glands, that ferry information throughout the body to regulate chemical reactions. This complex network of the hormones that specifically affect metabolism is referred to as the *peripheral metabolic pathway*. It includes chemical messengers that emanate from the fat mass, bones, muscle mass, gastrointestinal (GI) tract, pancreas, liver, endocrine glands, and blood components.

When we think of hormones, we often think of estrogen and testosterone: mood swings in adolescents and athletes on steroids, sex drive in men or hot flashes in middle-aged women. But hormones that regulate metabolism include a whole portfolio of different hormones, including some that are well known, such as insulin, and other, lesser-known hormones like adiponectin, leptin, glucagon, ghrelin, osteocalcin, oxyntomodulin, PYY, CCK, amylin, and various incretins such as GLP-1 and GIP. The hormone signals travel throughout the body and to the brain via this peripheral metabolic pathway, and in doing so they affect the higher metabolic centers in the brain to collectively influence our metabolism, weight, and appetite.

Every hormone communicates a very specific set of information. Imagine your body's hormones as functioning like a TV news team, where one commentator is an expert in politics, another covers the local weather, and yet another follows the latest celebrity news. Think of these reporters as being on air all day long, reporting the news and updating viewers.

Each hormone is emitted at a specific time and in a specific pattern. One might be released once a day, while another releases several times a day and still another several times an hour. Some hormones are secreted in pulses of microscopic droplets, like an IV drip. When each hormone is released, the bloodstream and nervous system carry it to receptors throughout the body whose job is to receive the hormonal signals, much like an antenna would.

The body's fat tissue, also known as fat mass, is actually the endocrine system's largest organ. Fat plays an enormously important role in regulating metabolism and influencing inflammation responses throughout the body. Collectively, the fat mass produces and secretes more hormones and bioactive chemicals, called *adipocytokines*, than any other endocrine gland. To date, scientists have identified more than eighty different influential proteins in the fat mass, including twenty-five hormones and numerous other chemical messengers.

Our fat tissue communicates with the rest of the body and the brain to regulate metabolism, appetite, and body weight—mainly by announcing its presence. When everything is functioning normally, hormones from the fat tissue tell the brain and other body parts how much we weigh, how well nourished we are, and how our body should respond to other endocrine hormonal signals essential to managing metabolism, weight, and appetite. Before the brain and body feel safe enough to carry out many nonessential functions—reproduction, for example—they must be convinced that the body has enough fat to survive a food emergency should one occur. Many weight problems are at least partly caused by abnormalities of certain hormones from the fat tissue.

Another extremely important hormone-producing system is the gastrointestinal system, which is thought to to manufacture more than forty individual hormones and peptides that enter the blood stream and nerve pathways. Collectively, these signals help regulate appetite, digestion, and absorption, and affect the body's rate of energy expenditure (calorie and body fat-burning processes).

Let's examine the role that several important hormones play in helping the metabolism function. Although it's not a comprehensive list, I hope it will help to illustrate the complexity of the metabolic system and the basics of how it works. (This is just for your information—there won't be a test on the material, I promise!)

STARS OF THE HORMONE SHOW
Insulin

Discovered in 1921, *insulin* is one of the major hormones that regulates metabolism. It is produced by the pancreas, which is located in the upper abdomen. Insulin's primary roles are to inform the brain that we are adequately nourished (have fuel on board), and to help transport glucose and proteins into the body cells so they can be used as energy.

Insulin "unlocks the door" to each cell so fuel can enter. (Note, however, that there are exceptions to this process: the brain, heart, and other vital organs can access glucose directly without requiring insulin.) Insulin's presence in the bloodstream signals to the brain and body that fuel is available, and it gives the body the green light to burn fuel that is in current circulation. It is generally produced in response to either a meal or snack, though it is also produced in smaller amounts during periods without food, such as at night or between meals when the liver releases its glucose stores to keep the blood supply steady.

Insulin can be measured with a routine lab test.

Glucagon

Glucagon was discovered in 1923. As insulin transports glucose into the cells after meals, the amount of glucose remaining in the bloodstream declines, which stimulates secretion of a second hormone from the pancreas: *glucagon*. Glucagon's role is to talk to the liver, which contains a reserve of glucose in the form of *glycogen*. Glucagon signals the liver to release a small amount of glucose into the bloodstream to "top off" the body's blood sugar between meals and keep it from dipping too low. Once the liver releases its stored glucose, the pancreas responds by secreting just enough insulin to transport any extra glucose into the cells for energy.

Scientists have recently found that glucagon, like insulin, influences the brain by providing critical information the brain needs to regulate blood sugar and metabolism. Together, glucagon and insulin maintain a steady glucose level within the body at all times, which is critical to normal metabolic function, thinking, mood, and energy. This is especially important because in normal circumstances, the brain uses nearly 100 percent glucose (which comes from dietary carbohydrates) for its own energy supply.

Glucagon, like insulin, can be measured with a routine lab test.

Leptin

Discovered in 1994, *leptin* is a powerful metabolism-regulating hormone primarily produced by fat tissue. Leptin travels through the bloodstream to receptor sites in the brain, liver, pancreas, bones, and nearly every type of body tissue. In doing so, it keeps the entire body informed and updated about how much a person weighs and whether he or she is carrying sufficient body fat to freely burn fat when the body needs energy.

The leptin signal is a major influencer of metabolism in the brain. Once received by the brain, if other reassuring signals are also present, the brain permits the appetite to regulate itself and allows the metabolism to function at full throttle. In other words, leptin from the peripheral system is required in order for the body's *satiety* cues to normalize—that is, in order for a person to feel satisfied after eating a meal. It also stimulates the metabolic rate to increase and body weight to balance. Leptin's other functions are to improve bone density, support the immune system, regulate thyroid levels, and

Fat Mass

Leptin is emitted from fat cells to inform the brain
and body of the status of the body's fat stores.

influence reproductive hormones (it strengthens fertility in both men and women).

Leptin levels can be measured clinically with a routine lab test.

Adiponectin

Discovered in 1996, *adiponectin* is another important hormone that is secreted by fat cells. Adiponectin sends signals to the muscle mass, and, to a lesser degree, the brain. Adiponectin is a powerful "insulin sensitizer," meaning it increases muscle cells' sensitivity to insulin. This in turn helps insulin move glucose out of the bloodstream and into the cells more easily. Adiponectin also stimulates metabolism in the body's muscle mass at rest and during exercise and reduces total body inflammation, particularly in the blood vessels. This means that when the fat mass—the very same fat that popular culture proclaims is hazardous to good health—communicates normally, it actually plays a vital role in helping the body burn energy and in keeping blood vessels free of inflammation, which can prevent strokes, diabetes, and heart attacks.

Adiponectin levels can be measured clinically with a routine blood test.

Gut Hormones

Discovered in 1902, gut hormones are very important players in metabolism, appetite, and weight regulation.

The incretins, including GLP-1, announce food intake
to the brain and body.

JUST THE FACTS

Leptin-Adiponectin Ratio

Researchers have explored whether the ratio of leptin in the body relative to adiponectin may predict a person's risk of strokes, diabetes, heart attacks, and other catastrophic events. The higher the person's leptin level relative to the amount of adiponectin they emit, the greater, some experts believe, the person's risk is for these types of problems.

However, recent studies suggest that adiponectin levels may more accurately predict these potential health risks and hazards when measured alone, regardless of leptin levels.

Incretins, which include GIP and GLP-1, are one group of hormones emitted by the gastrointestinal tract (or gut). Other gut hormones include ghrelin, PYY, oxyntomodulin, and many more.

The incretin group of gut hormones helps regulate communication between the gut and the brain, telling the brain when and what a person is eating. These hormones control the pace at which food moves through the stomach and small intestine, and the pace at which nutrients, including glucose, are absorbed and released into the bloodstream. Incretins also help the pancreas balance insulin and glucagon levels to maintain a consistent level of glucose in the bloodstream after a person eats.

By informing and assuring the body and the brain about food availability, all the gut hormones play a major role in regulating the central metabolic pathway, appetite receptor satiety cues, and the metabolic rate.

Currently, most gut hormones—including incretins—are not usually measured in a clinical setting, but many are routinely measured in research settings. Recently, we have been able to measure GLP-1, GIP, PYY and ghrelin clinically through specialty laboratories. GLP-1 levels before and after a meal can be helpful for detecting malfunction of this hormone balance. GLP-1 levels should at least double after a meal and many patients with obesity have deficiency of this hormone before eating and show a failure to increase after eating a full meal.

More on Ghrelin

Discovered in 1999, *ghrelin*, one of the gut hormones, is produced primarily by the tissue along the lower curve of the stomach. Ghrelin informs the brain when the body's short-term fuel supply has run out between meals and signals that food is needed. This is why ghrelin carries the popular nickname: the "hunger hormone."

Ghrelin is the only peripheral hormone and one of the few chemicals in the body that blocks rather than stimulates the metabolism, blocking the signals to the central pathway. During ghrelin surges, metabolism slows down and appetite increases. If ghrelin fails to decline after a person eats and its baseline remains elevated, that person's weight will usually increase. Ghrelin also opposes the action of all of the hormones that turn the metabolism "on" and the appetite "down." Whereas other gut hormones (like GLP-1, oxyntomodulin, and PYY) stimulate the metabolic rate, calm the appetite receptors, and lower body weight, high ghrelin levels do the opposite.

Total ghrelin levels can be measured clinically with a routine blood test. I used to ask scientists if as a clinician I had to worry about ghrelin causing problems in my patients. Most often the response was "no because ghrelin is a short-term hormone and as soon as a meal is consumed it drops and moves out of the way." But in my practice, similar to what has been observed in research studies, ghrelin can easily become a long-term hormone in people with metabolic dysfunction and can be very much a part of their metabolic problem. I have found it can be helpful to measure pre-and post-meal ghrelin levels, as ghrelin should suppress within an hour of eating a meal under normal circumstances. Many of our patients show a lack of ghrelin suppression post prandially, which means their ghrelin does not drop normally after eating, ultimately contributing to their weight problem.

Amylin

Discovered in 1988, *amylin* is a hormone produced by the pancreas that helps the brain "see" the leptin signal. These two hormones are found to work synergistically to stimulate the metabolic system. Therefore, amylin has a major role in enabling and influencing metabolic rate and satiety. Like leptin, amylin helps the brain regulate the function of the thyroid, ovaries, testicles, and several other glands. Like incretins, amylin helps regulate the pace at which nutrients empty from the stomach into the small intestine and then into the bloodstream, and it helps regulate the pancreas's glucagon response to prevent glucose levels in the blood from increasing above normal ranges.

Currently, amylin levels cannot be measured in a clinical setting, but can be measured in research settings. By 2016, amylin levels may be made available clinically. Similar to ghrelin, GLP-1 and PYY, amylin levels vary before and after meals, but in contrast to ghrelin and similar to GLP-1 and PYY, amylin surges within an hour of consuming a meal in a normal situation. Since it's secreting along with insulin, if insulin levels are high, amylin levels can be high and if insulin levels are low, amylin levels are low.

Alpha-Melanocyte Stimulating Hormone

Abbreviated MSH, melanocyte stimulating hormone is the only hormone we are mentioning in this section that is produced primarily by the brain, or specifically by the pituitary gland rather than the peripheral system. This key hormone helps carry an important signal to the satiety receptors in the brain that regulate appetite and to the receptors responsible for weight regulation, energy expenditure, and insulin production. It has other actions throughout the body, including an influence on skin pigmentation in Caucasians. This hormone is produced from another pituitary hormone, adrenocorticotropic hormone, or ACTH. ACTH is most commonly known to stimulate cortisol production from the adrenal gland but few people, even doctors, are aware of its other powerful role in metabolism.

Currently, alpha MSH and ACTH levels can be routinely measured clinically.

THAT'S THE GANG

The hormones you've just learned about are some of the most important players along the peripheral metabolic pathway. The signals they send make their way to the brain and its central metabolic pathway, where the information is processed and acted upon.

Key Metabolic Hormones

FUNCTIONS	MALFUNCTIONS
Leptin	**Low Leptin / Leptin Resistance**
Informs the brain of body weight and fat status Increases metabolism Increases satiety Regulates reproductive and thyroid hormones	Decreases metabolic rate Decreases reproductive and thyroid hormones Decreases satiety Increases hunger Weight gain
Insulin	**Insulin Resistance**
Informs the brain the body is nourished Transports glucose and protein into cells Builds muscle Prevents diabetes	Weight-loss resistance Increases belly fat Sugar cravings Fatigue / low energy
Adiponectin	**Low Adiponectin**
Increases metabolism Increases insulin sensitivity Decreases inflammation	Increases risk for diabetes, stroke, and heart attack Weight loss resistance Increases inflammation
GLP-1	**GLP-1 Malfunction**
Informs the brain of food supply Controls the pace of food transport and absorption Increases satiety Increases metabolic rate Decreases belly fat	Decreases satiety Increases hunger Weight gain Increases belly fat
Ghrelin	**High Ghrelin***
Increases hunger Decreases satiety Decreases metabolism Affects fertility	Weight gain Weight-loss resistance Increases hunger *Also increases NPY and AgRP

Metabolic Conditions

Pre-Diabetes	Diabetes
Diagnostic criteria:	**Diagnostic criteria:**
HbA1C: 5.7 - 6.3	HbA1C: 6.4 +
Fasting glucose: 100 - 125	Fasting glucose: 126 +
Common signs and symptoms:	**Common signs and symptoms:**
Decreased metabolic rate	Decreased metabolic rate
Weight-loss resistance	Weight-loss resistance
Weight gain	Weight gain
Sugar cravings	Sugar cravings
Acanthosis nigricans	Acanthosis nigricans
Stretch marks	Stretch marks
	Increased thirst
	Increased hunger
	Increased urination
	Changes in vision
	Nerve pain

Metabolic Syndrome

A combination of three or more of the following:

- Abnormal cholesterol panel such as:
  Increased Triglycerides
  Increased LDL particles
  Decreased HDL

- Increased blood pressure

- Increased abdominal circumference:
  35" or more in women
  40" or more in men

- Increased glucose or insulin

Chapter 4

Brain is Boss

THE FOUR-DOOR SYSTEM

The *central metabolic pathway* is the portion of the feedback loop that consists of the brain and the nervous system. It receives incoming signals from the peripheral metabolic pathway, then processes and interprets those signals to determine whether to give a green, yellow, or red light to the body's metabolic processes. This action ultimately determines whether the body will lose, maintain, or gain weight. For simplicity's sake, I describe the central metabolic pathway as a four-door system. There are four *mandatory* doors that must open in order for the body to let go of excess weight. When glitches occur along the pathway, keeping the doors from opening normally, they can cause body fat accumulation, difficulty losing excess weight, reduced metabolism, and a heightened appetite.

Door Number One

Door One, the first door of the central metabolic pathway, is called the *arcuate nucleus* (ARC). The ARC involves the hypothalamus, the body's highest-level gland, which governs daily operation of the body's other glands. The ARC is the entry point through which messengers coming from the peripheral metabolic pathway arrive at the brain, where their signals are processed.

The neurons (specialized cells) within the ARC not only permeate the hypothalamus but also extend and transmit information into the next gland down in the hierarchy, the pituitary gland, which also directs other glands throughout the body.

The ARC neurons produce two specific chemicals called neurotransmitters—I call them "guards"—that play a major role at Door One. These chemicals are called *neuropeptide Y* (NPY), and *agouti-related protein* (AgRP). NPY and AgRP are two of the body's most powerful chemicals when it comes to blocking metabolic function. When they are elevated, they send starvation signals through the brain and body, stimulating appetite and slowing metabolism.

The "Four Doors" of the Central Metabolic Pathway

A Normally Functioning System

A Malfunctioning System

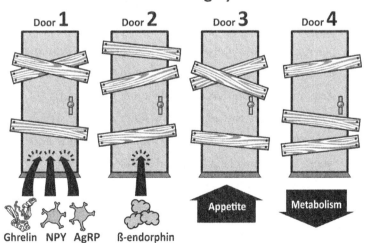

©2015 Emily Cooper, M.D.

By default, both NPY and AgRP remain on high alert (in an elevated position), assuming that the body is in a malnourished and low body-weight state, until hormones and other messengers from the peripheral metabolic pathway successfully prove that the body weighs enough and has sufficient fuel. In other words, for our own protection, NPY and AgRP need a "coast is clear" signal from the body to allow their levels to drop.

The problem is that, as mentioned earlier, the NPY levels of a patient with anorexia and a BMI of 12 and a patient with obesity and a BMI over 60 can be the same even though only one of the patients is actually starving, because glitches in the feedback loop can create an erroneous perception of starvation. When NPY and AgRP remain elevated in this way, the brain thinks it's not safe to allow the metabolic process to proceed to Door Two.

Important signals are received at the ARC. Leptin signals from the body's fat tissue communicate whether a person has sufficient body mass. Insulin signals from the pancreas inform the brain that the body is in a nourished state and therefore has access to food. Glucose, GLP-1, PYY, and other messengers also send the ARC signals, providing information on nutritional status and body weight and influencing NPY and AgRP levels.

When incoming signals convince the ARC that the body has sufficient weight and nourishment, a green light is given to allow for metabolically stimulating reactions to proceed. NPY and AgRP levels are allowed to sharply decline, opening Door One and removing the obstacles to opening Door Two.

NPY can be measured clinically with a routine lab test. Usually AgRP can only be measured in research settings at this time but specialty laboratories are soon making this important test available clinically.

Door Number Two

Door Two is located in the pituitary gland. This is where the precursor hormone *propiomelanacortin* (POMC) converts to *adrenocorticotropic hormone* (ACTH), which in turn produces the metabolism-stimulating hormone *melanocyte stimulating hormone* (MSH). So, opening Door Two is really the process of converting one hormone to another: POMC to ACTH, and ACTH to MSH. Once MSH is available, there are not too many additional processes needed to allow the metabolism to increase, weight to drop, and the appetite to settle down.

However, because the body really wants to protect us in case of famine, it's not easy to open Door Two. The neurotransmitter *gamma-aminobutyric acid* (GABA) is the primary guard at this door: it puts the brakes on chemical reactions throughout the body to keep them from going too fast. A drop in NPY, however, causes GABA to drop, thus allowing Door Two to open and POMC to convert to MSH. Interestingly, this door has a natural braking mechanism that makes it operate similar to a saloon door. Once it pushes open, it creates a counter momentum to slam shut. This happens because POMC also converts to b-endorphin, which can actually shutdown the ACTH and MSH production. Endurance athletes and people on extreme diets often have abnormally high b-endorphin levels, which can keep Door Two closing repeatedly.

ACTH and MSH can be measured clinically with routine lab tests. GABA and POMC cannot be measured clinically at this time. And it's not clear whether testing for b-endorphin reliably reflects brain concentrations.

Door Number Three

Door Three is comprised of the *melanocortin 3 receptors* (MC3Rs) located in the hypothalamus and limbic areas (memory, motivation, and emotion centers) of the brain. MC3Rs control our appetite, affecting our interest in food and level of satisfaction after eating. Door Three opens when the newly formed MSH, produced from opening Door Two, connects correctly with the MC3Rs. Receptors like the MC3Rs are like antennas that receive hormone signals, in this case MSH. You can also think of receptors and hormones as jigsaw puzzle pieces, the receptors having openings that the hormones fit into perfectly. When the MC3Rs detect the MSH and 'open' successfully, the body experiences normal hunger levels and normal satisfaction levels after eating a meal. In other words, when MC3Rs work properly, people don't think about how much to eat or whether they are done eating—it's very natural and automatic.

But as in other parts of the process, there can be glitches with this step. If MSH signals are too low or if MSH has a problem connecting properly with the MC3Rs, the body is not likely to experience normal hunger and satiety cues. Instead, depending on how weak the signal is at the MC3Rs, there may be a preoccupation with food, excessive hunger, and lack of satisfaction even after a normal meal.

Genetic testing for MC3R malfunction is not yet available clinically.

Door Number Four

Door Four is located throughout the brain. *Melanocortin 4 receptors* (MC4Rs) also receive the signals from MSH which essentially activates the MC4Rs. By doing so, they regulate metabolism and ultimately determine whether body weight will increase, decrease, or stay the same. In essence, MC4Rs regulate the body's weight-set point. This door opens when MSH fits precisely into the MC4Rs. At this point, the body receives a final "all clear" signal to increase metabolic rate and reduce body weight.

However, things can go wrong at the MC4Rs. For example, if ghrelin levels are very high, and if the AgRP from Door One hasn't dropped far enough, MSH can be blocked from connecting with and activating the MC4Rs, which means the body won't receive the green light it's waiting for, signaling that it's safe to let go of extra body weight.

In addition to problems with elevated ghrelin and AgRP and insufficient MSH levels, some patients have a genetic condition causing half of their MC4R's to malfunction.

Genetic mutations of the MC4Rs are handed down from one parent, and each child has a 50% chance of inheriting the condition. It is most often associated with early-onset obesity in childhood or adolescence. These specific genetic glitches are present in about 2-4% of the population with obesity.

Genetic testing for MC4R genetic mutation is clinically available but very expensive and not usually covered by insurance.

CHECKS AND BALANCES

The metabolic signals that flow along the central pathway in the brain communicate back to the body, relaying what the brain thinks of the body's overall nutritional status. The peripheral pathway messages, then, communicate back to the central pathway. If all goes smoothly, this feedback loop is a well-oiled machine that keeps the appetite calm and the body weight balanced in a normal range. But if the feedback loop encounters a glitch, that one glitch can lead to another in a domino effect that causes higher body weight, slower metabolic function, and often appetite malfunction.

Communication between the pathways is instantaneous and dynamic. Hormones from the peripheral metabolic pathway can alter their signals, depending upon reciprocal signals from the brain. In turn, the brain interprets the incoming hormonal signals and instructs the central metabolic pathway on how much fuel it should let the body burn. By communicating back and forth in this fashion, neither the brain nor the body permits the other to compromise the body's perceived nutritional status.

You might think of this communication system as being similar to the way a couple with a joint checking account might manage their account balance. A certain amount of money comes in each month, but many different ways of spending it exist: cash withdrawals, checks, online bill payments, electronic transfers, and debit or credit card purchases. Either partner (or both) can use the account simultaneously—which means that without a system of checks and balances, both partners could withdraw as much money as they wanted, with potentially disastrous consequences.

The metabolic feedback loop functions similarly, allowing each partner—in this analogy, the peripheral and central pathways—to know the account balance and make adjustments accordingly so neither partner depletes the account. The fat mass, digestive tract, organs, glands, receptor sites, blood components, and other elements of the peripheral system communicate to the brain and make adjustments instantaneously, preserving the energy balance they perceive as appropriate.

WRAP-UP

When leptin, insulin, and other chemical signals from the peripheral metabolic pathway convince the brain that the body is not in nutritional danger, and if no other factors interfere, the central metabolic pathway is put into motion, beginning with NPY and AgRP levels dropping to open Door One. When Door One opens wide enough, usually all of the other doors open, and the metabolism is free to burn incoming fuel, body weight balances normally, and the appetite is calmed. This is what happens routinely in normal-weight people with normal metabolisms—and, as unbelievable as it may sound, when an overweight person's metabolic system has rebooted itself and starts working correctly, this will happen for them as well, and they will automatically begin to lose their excess weight.

As tough as it is to deal with weight problems, when glitches in the metabolic pathway occur, the body is really just doing its job: protecting us from perceived harm by storing more fat.

CHAPTER 5

Food Intake and Utilization

THE METABOLISM CONSISTS OF all of the biological and chemical processes that convert the food we eat into the energy our body needs to function well. The body must coordinate thousands of simultaneous metabolic activities just so the heart can beat and the brain can work.

Whether we are active or at rest, our metabolism is always hard at work managing our fuel and energy balance. Metabolism is a constant process; it may slow down or speed up, but it never stops. It is the sum total of all reactions in the body: it allows the body to convert fuel and fuel stores into energy, which, enables activities as basic as breathing and as complex as running a marathon.

Our metabolism depends on regular fuel intake to stabilize the body's nutritional status and make energy available. The body accomplishes this by following four steps: foraging (or innate eating), digestion, absorption, and finally utilization. Utilization involves converting nutrients into energy to use in one of three ways (this is called *energy partitioning*): for immediate use to power the body or brain; for later use (kept as fat stores); and for building and repairing structural body tissue like muscles, tendons, bone, and skin.

STEP 1: FORAGING—PEOPLE DO IT TOO

The first metabolic activity is *foraging*. Of course, we're familiar with animals' innate foraging behavior: bears rummage through the woods for berries, and squirrels dig for buried nuts. However, we tend to give little thought to humans having similar eating behaviors. Innate eating is not dictated by a clock or schedule; rather, it's largely driven by hormonal activity among the brain, fat, muscles, bones, gastrointestinal tract, organs, and other parts of the body that we may not even associate with our appetite.

As I mentioned in Chapter 3, the metabolism is regulated by a complex feedback loop whereby the body and the brain communicate through hormone signals. These hormones impact the appetite receptors that direct our innate eating experience. Various communication centers throughout the body inform the brain and body about the amount of food and the type of nutrients that are needed as fuel.

This inner wisdom may cause us to desire or crave foods that we innately know contain the nutrients we need in the quantities we need them. How do we know this? Because our ancestors' survival depended on knowing what nutrients certain foods contained, and their evolved eating habits have influenced our DNA.

Let's say you develop a distinct craving for tomatoes. You decide to make spaghetti with red sauce and eat it for dinner that night and as lunch the next day. If this satisfies your taste for tomatoes, you may not crave them again for a while. Maybe it's just that you knew it would taste good—but it's also possible that your body needed to obtain a specific nutrient found in tomatoes, and that's what caused you to crave them. Once you eat some tomatoes, the nutritional need is met, and your appetite for tomatoes may go away for a while.

These types of cravings can be incredibly specific. We're all familiar with stories of pregnant women who develop a taste for pickles or some other unusual food. Sometimes people even yearn for foods they've never had before. When this happens, it's likely that the brain is acting upon information that's been passed down through generations genetically.

Food as a Distraction

When the metabolism is functioning normally, food generally isn't overly attractive—a bag of chips in the cupboard or donuts at the office should not call to you to the point of distraction. However, if the metabolism is not functioning normally and appetite receptors are not firing properly, food—especially high-sugar, high-fat, or high-calorie foods—may relentlessly beckon to you. While someone with normal appetite receptor function may pick up a handful of potato chips and move on, someone with a malfunctioning feedback loop will probably be distracted by the chips and will have to wage an internal battle in order to ignore the urge to eat all of them.

When is Enough Enough?

I refer to satisfaction as coming from two places: the brain and the stomach. Frequently, people with a metabolic problem might stop eating only because everyone around them has stopped or because their stomach feels overly full. They don't stop eating because their brain senses they have had enough to eat and they feel satisfied. Because of this, the eating experience of people with metabolic issues often feels urgent, a feeling that can lead to faster eating and greater food intake. This happens because brain receptors (MC3Rs and even MC4Rs) aren't registering the food intake and, therefore, fail to signal that the meal is over.

Another common symptom of a malfunctioning metabolism is feeling the need to think about what was eaten throughout the day before deciding what to eat next. Conversely, people with a normally functioning metabolic pathway never feel a need to think about what they have previously eaten. They eat what and how much they want or need each time they are hungry. Then they move on, never looking back. Their brain senses that it's time to stop eating, and their stomach feels satisfied and comfortable. This is why people with normally functioning metabolisms end their meals. It's a simple concept, but one that is foreign to many people who struggle with a malfunctioning metabolism and excess body weight.

Elizabeth had a lifelong struggle with her weight, which eventually led her to undergo gastric bypass surgery years ago. Although she initially experienced considerable weight loss after her surgery, her weight later steadily—and uncontrollably—increased. Out of desperation, Elizabeth asked her surgeon if a band could be put around her tiny remaining stomach pouch. When she found this was not possible, she felt completely hopeless. After enrolling in a medically supervised diet program with little success, she came to see me as a last resort.

When I tested Elizabeth, I found that her metabolic pathway was not working correctly and that her blood sugar was plummeting to very low levels immediately after she ate. After implementing medical treatment to address these underlying metabolic problems, her body weight decreased and her appetite normalized—without dieting.

"I used to be a secret junk and sugar eater," Elizabeth shared. "Now, I'm really not. It's not a conscious decision or that I'm trying to reform. I just don't want to drag a pie home anymore. I can just get a piece of pie if I want to. No one is saying I can't. There are no more rules for the first time in my life."

Elizabeth's observations highlight the impact of a faulty metabolic feedback loop on appetite and body weight. When the loop is realigned and the metabolic signals make their way successfully to the end of the central metabolic pathway, appetite and body weight respond automatically. If Elizabeth's eating behaviors and weight struggles of the past were behavioral rather than medical, how could a lifelong problem have changed so dramatically in a matter of weeks, solely through medical treatment?

Biology vs. Behavior

Scientists have found that cues for eating and moving are significantly affected by biological factors arising from the peripheral and central metabolic pathways. While not all of my patients with weight issues have problems with eating cues, the vast majority has a heightened appetite response, impaired satisfaction after meals, and frequent preoccupation with food. It is very important to note, however, that this is a *biological* problem caused by glitches in the metabolic feedback loop, not a *behavioral* problem.

My patients often tell me they can't have tempting food in their house or they'll eat it.

"I'm a smart person!" Helen complained. "I'm running a company. So why can't I be in charge of this? It's the one area of my life where I don't understand why I can't achieve my goals. I'm competent in every other area of my life."

"I never feel satisfied unless I eat four pounds of pasta," Christine admitted.

"An hour after finishing a large meal," Dan told me, "I'm craving Mexican food—I'm starving."

Although these responses are symptoms of underlying biological issues, people often blame them on lack of control and refer to indulging such cravings as binge eating, stress eating, emotional eating, or boredom eating. After treating hundreds of patients with appetite issues, however, it has become clear to me that these symptoms are actually caused by short circuits affecting a portion (or portions) of the metabolic pathway. The appetite receptors are not receiving the message that the body is adequately fueled, and therefore they are not allowing the appetite to calm down.

Once appetite cues are unbalanced, is there any hope of regaining normal innate eating habits? In my experience, the answer is "YES." Remarkably, with treatment targeted at improving the signaling throughout the metabolic pathway, symptoms can dissipate within days. Many of my patients report that for the first time in decades— or even for the first time ever—they actually experience "what it feels like to be normal" in terms of hunger, food interest, and satisfaction.

Like Elizabeth, patients who have regained metabolic balance report that food used to call out to them. "If I was at a bakery and saw some delicious-looking cake, I might buy the entire cake," one patient said. "But now I walk past the bakery and I'm not as interested. I might buy one piece of cake and feel free to enjoy it at a normal pace without feeling desperate or guilty, or without craving more." Other patients have said that even when they're enjoying their favorite meal and there is food left on their plate, they can now feel completely satisfied and naturally stop eating.

Indeed, most patients tell me that having normal appetite regulation—what people with normal metabolic function take for granted—is "an incredibly freeing experience."

Food Indecision

Although it's less common, metabolic impairment can also cause decreased appetite or an absence of appetite. Patients with this kind of metabolic issue tend to struggle with making food choices, either having trouble deciding between foods or feeling that nothing looks good. People whose metabolic pathway is working properly, in contrast, usually know what they want and can make a decision fairly quickly.

People with impaired metabolic function may experience a great deal of indecision, often opening cabinets or standing in front of the refrigerator door, eating this or that or this *and* that, in an effort to satisfy their appetite. Some cope with their indecision by sticking to a fixed eating schedule, thereby avoiding the uncertainty of not knowing what to eat or feeling like they are not in control of what they eat.

I have observed that it is less common to experience an unusually decreased or absent appetite than it is to experience an overly increased appetite—but both issues are equally indicative of metabolic malfunction.

STEP 2: DIGESTION

Although we often associate *digestion* with the stomach, the digestive process actually begins in the mouth, where enzymes in the saliva begin breaking food down into components the body can absorb. When we chew, the body activates additional enzymes further down the gastrointestinal (GI) tract that help prepare the body to absorb the incoming nutrients, ready the pancreas for insulin production, and activate hormones in the gut that tell the brain we are eating, which is what makes us feel satiated.

The food then travels down the esophagus and into the stomach. Here, the *stretch receptors*, which are part of the nervous system, sense when the stomach is full. Meanwhile, a variety of hormones and enzymes coordinate the digestive process, helping the stomach break down the food, assisting absorption, and communicating to the rest of the body that we are eating.

Eventually, acids and enzymes in the stomach transform the food into liquid, making it easier for the body to absorb nutrients. The liquefied food then enters the small intestine—a narrow, 20-plus-foot-long tube that snakes between the stomach and large intestine—and the small intestine finishes digesting the food, breaking the macronutrients down into their smallest components: glucose and other sugars, amino acids, fatty acids, and micronutrients (vitamins and minerals).

People often complain that they feel bloated after eating. This frequently happens when hormonal malfunctions cause the stomach to empty at irregular rates. Incretins (the hormones in the lower GI tract that we discussed in Chapter 3) regulate the pace at which the stomach empties, but when there are deficiencies of these hormones our brain doesn't sense satiety, and the stomach can empty into the small intestine too rapidly. Because we don't feel full, we may increase the pace and quantity of our food intake, causing the stomach to become overly distended. Without normally functioning satiety cues, we begin to rely on this bloated feeling to know we've had enough to eat. In contrast, for a person with normal metabolic function, satiety cues are sensed in the brain first, followed by the stomach.

STEP 3: ABSORPTION

Tiny "fingers," or *villi*, that line the walls of the small intestine transport sugars, amino acids, fatty acids, vitamins, and minerals out of the intestine and into the bloodstream, which carries the nutrients throughout the body for utilization. When the metabolism is operating normally, the pace of nutrient absorption is perfectly matched to pancreas insulin production by hormones from the brain and GI tract, ensuring optimal nutrient processing and utilization. When the metabolism is malfunctioning, however, these hormones may be non-operational or deficient. This can make the pace of nutrient absorption irregular or too rapid, causing a mismatch of glucose with insulin and creating a suboptimal environment for nutrient processing and utilization.

STEP 4: UTILIZATION

When the body is well-tuned and feels secure that it has enough food and body mass, it will distribute absorbed nutrients based on the needs of its various parts and their functions.

A healthy metabolism paces itself, speeding up or slowing down fuel utilization based on the energy demands the body places upon it. This helps to explain why some people maintain a normal weight for their entire life—they have a healthy metabolism that manages their weight for them, keeping them in a normal range.

Chapter 6

Welcome to Metabolism 101

METABOLIC RATES

Metabolic rate refers to the number of calories the body burns per minute to complete tasks at hand. The body's metabolic rate is continually set and adjusted by the metabolic feedback loop based on the brain and body's perception of body weight, food availability, and what activities are being performed.

The ability to measure metabolism by what is called *indirect calorimetry* was discovered in 1780. By the 1940s, scientists studying metabolism and obesity were routinely measuring metabolic response to various diets. Today's equipment is streamlined, comfortable for the patient, and much easier to use than the equipment used seventy years ago, but the concept behind it is the same: metabolism rates are determined by measuring the body's "exhaust" in a patient's exhaled breath. This exhaust contains oxygen and carbon dioxide and, based on the volume of each, the number of calories and the type of fuel burned (protein, carbohydrate or fat) can be closely estimated.

Basal Metabolism

The majority of the calories we consume are burned while our body is running at its *basal metabolic rate* (BMR), the background burn rate at which it operates while we're sleeping. You would be surprised how much energy we expend lying flat on our back. Keeping the brain running, heart beating, blood flowing, lungs breathing, liver and kidneys functioning, and bowels moving—maintaining all the activities essential to life—requires a tremendous number of calories, and the body saves its heavy lifting for the night shift, when few other energy demands exist. For example, we grow and repair injured body parts while we're sleeping—whether it's tendons, ligaments, bones, organs, or skin. This is one reason why it's vital that we not skimp on sleep: it's critical for completing the metabolic processes of regeneration.

Resting Metabolism & Daily Metabolism Rates

The rate at which the metabolism operates when it's resting is higher than our basal metabolic rate, because it has to accommodate the additional energy we expend while awake and alert.

The *daily metabolic rate* differs from the *resting metabolic rate* because it includes the additional energy we expend when we're involved in our daily activities—showering, eating, moving around, caring for our children, driving to work, and so on.

Resting Metabolism: Fed State

The four hours or so that it takes to eat and digest a meal make up what we call the body's *fed metabolic state*. During this time, nutrients flow out of food and into the bloodstream, then the body divides the fuel up to either expend immediately or store for later. In its fed state, the body processes and burns what is immediately on hand rather than stored fat. While the body digests food, the metabolic rate raises about 10 percent above where it operates when we have not eaten. This effect of food upon the metabolic rate is referred to as its *thermogenic* effect.

Resting Metabolism: Fasting State

Beginning about four hours after we eat, after the main work of digestion is complete and the energy and nutrients from a meal have been apportioned, the resting metabolism re-enters its *fasting state*. Glucose no longer flows out of the food and into the bloodstream; instead, the liver's glycogen releases glucose into the bloodstream to balance blood sugar levels. The bloodstream then carries that glucose to the body cells, where it becomes the main source of energy between meals.

In its resting state, the metabolism normally burns equal amounts of carbohydrates (glucose) and fat, plus a very small amount of protein. If we don't eat enough carbohydrates, the body burns more protein because it can convert protein to carbohydrates. Since the brain must have glucose to operate normally, carbohydrates are essential for normal mood and brain function. The body cannot convert fats to carbohydrates, so if it needs more carbs, it takes proteins from the muscles and immune system to supply the needed energy. This results in muscle breakdown and reduced immune function.

Exercising Metabolism

Muscles usually can't absorb glucose from the bloodstream without help from the hormone insulin. However, during exercise only, the muscle cells—which are the most

JUST THE FACTS

Many misconceptions exist about exercise and burning fat. The fat the body burns during exercise consists primarily of liquid droplets of fat stored in the muscles, not body fat from adipose tissue.

metabolically active cells in the body—have an additional way to access circulating glucose that doesn't require insulin. Muscle cells store carbohydrates as glycogen and fats as triglycerides in the form of liquid fuel droplets. The muscle cells can access immediate energy from these fuel droplets during exercise rather than having to wait for energy to arrive from elsewhere in the body. By exercise I'm referring to any continuous motion that challenges the body, such as a jog, a swim, a bike ride, or even gardening or a brisk walk. The muscle cells utilize whatever glycogen and triglycerides exist inside of them, and then, if necessary, they replenish themselves with glucose from the bloodstream to tank up energy stores for future use.

Regular, consistent exercisers and endurance athletes store more glycogen in their muscles than non-athletes. They need this extra fuel to meet the strenuous demands that they place on their body. About three hours of carbohydrate energy are stored in a trained athlete's muscles. In contrast, sedentary people store only enough energy in their muscles to react to immediate demands or emergencies. As you will learn in the next chapter, if someone has metabolic problems that include insulin resistance, glycogen stores may be diminished due to the difficulty glucose has getting into their muscle cells.

WORKING HARD, GETTING NOWHERE

Like appetite, the impetus to move—scientifically called *locomotive activity*—is also directly affected by the status of the metabolic pathway. For example, high levels of ghrelin, insulin resistance, and adiponectin malfunction have been found to affect the muscles' ability to store and access energy. In animal studies, forcibly increasing ghrelin levels in an animal's body has been shown to lead to a reduction of *ad lib locomotion*—meaning that the animal becomes sluggish and reduces its movement. When this problem is reversed in the laboratory and ghrelin levels return to normal, the animal immediately regains its movement and begins to exercise.[1]

Humans are no different than laboratory mice in this regard: we directly respond to the body's perceptions of our energy balance. As you may recall from Chapter 3, the body's reaction to the perception of starvation can

1. I.D. Blum, Z. Patterson, R. Khazall, et al., "Reduced Anticipatory Locomotor Responses to Scheduled Meals in Ghrelin Receptor Deficient Mice," *Neuroscience* (December 8, 2009), doi: 10.1016/j.neuroscience.2009.08.009, PMCID: PMC2996828.

often be as strong as its reaction to actual sta
duction in movement is part of the body's atte
serve energy and store fat for protection.

Over time, people with hormonal imbalances can feel tired, hungry, and eventually exhausted. Exercise, in particular, can become increasingly difficult, even uncomfortable. Not surprisingly, this can cause some people to become inactive. However, in spite of these serious challenges, many of my patients who struggle with weight issues are extremely athletic.

Meg has been an avid cyclist her entire life and commutes to work by bike several times a week—but in spite of her athleticism, she struggles with obesity, insulin resistance, and other metabolic issues. "I ride my bike all year round," she said. "I know I'm stronger and more fit than many of the cyclists I see on the road, but they are always passing me, especially on the hills. It's really frustrating and demoralizing. I'm a serious athlete, but I don't look or perform like one in spite of all my efforts."

Meg is in good company. In general, many of my patients are exercising far more and being more careful about their food intake than normal-weight people. I see some patients who have the fitness level of a competitive endurance athlete, but their performance doesn't even come close to reflecting their level of fitness. Due to the excess weight they are carrying, they expend a significant portion of their energy merely moving their body forward—which means that they are likely to be slower than their normal-weight competitors, regardless of their fitness level.

Thus many people become sedentary not because they don't want to exercise or because they're inherently lazy, but because exercise is much harder for them than it is for people with a normal metabolism. When metabolic hormones are balanced, people increase their locomotion; when their metabolism is blocked by hormonal imbalances, they decrease locomotion. The desire to be inactive is a biological and hormonal response, not simply a lifestyle choice.

A normally functioning metabolism can rev up or down as the situation warrants. For example, resting metabolic rate increases after exercise to help the body perform additional tasks, such as strengthening tissues and repairing micro-tears, in a process called *afterburn*. During afterburn, the resting metabolism increases slightly for a time period that can range from minutes to days, depending on the type of workout the person has engaged in. With an impaired metabolism, afterburn may not take place, which can lead to the metabolism rate actually decreasing in the hours after exercise in an attempt to compensate for a falsely perceived energy deficiency.

While many people with metabolism problems are avid athletes and feel great when they exercise, it makes sense that some people with metabolic problems complain of being tired after exercise and not experiencing the "exercise high" that many other people describe.

"I feel tired after exercise. I feel like I'm struggling through it," some of my patients complain. Others tell me, "I exercise first thing in the morning to get it out of the way because I hate it" or "People say exercise is refreshing, but I never feel invigorated afterward."

DOCTOR, PLEASE CHECK MY THYROID!

So many people with a weight problem think they might have a sluggish thyroid gland. And while the thyroid gland does affect metabolism, and low thyroid levels, called hypothyroidism, are fairly common, thyroid disease is not responsible for all the complaints we hear about feeling tired or gaining weight. Patients are often frustrated when they have these symptoms and know something has to be wrong—yet doctors check their thyroid and say everything is fine. But other metabolic conditions could be the issue. Problems with metabolism can not only cause similar symptoms as hypothyroidism but they can also affect thyroid levels, making thyroid lab tests confusing and difficult to interpret, even for doctors.

When metabolic glitches trigger the brain to wrongly think the body is starving, these glitches can also affect your thyroid levels. That's why it's always important to review your numbers with your healthcare provider. Keep in mind that the thyroid gland only makes as much thyroid hormone as the brain tells it to make, so the *brain* is in charge of the thyroid levels. In hypothyroidism in spite of the brain telling the thyroid to make thyroid hormone, the thyroid can't respond because it's diseased. But in the case of metabolism glitches, the brain perceives starvation so it won't tell the thyroid to make more hormone because it wants to keep the levels low to conserve energy and store fat for protection.

Hypothyroid
- High TSH (from brain)
- Low thyroid levels (T4, T3)

Metabolic Glitches
- Low or normal TSH (from brain)
- Low thyroid levels (T4, T3)

The following illustrations show a normally functioning thyroid pathway and one that is impacted due to metabolic glitches. In contrast, in hypothyroidism due to thyroid disease, the TSH level remains high and the T4 and T3 levels are low, not due to leptin or ghrelin imbalances but due to the fact that the gland itself is diseased and therefore cannot produce thyroid hormone.

The thyroid hormone pathway

Hypothalamus

TRH
Thyrotropin-releasing Hormone

Pituitary

TSH
Thyroid Stimulating Hormone

Leptin

T4

Thyroid Gland

Free
T3

©2015 Emily Cooper, M.D.

The thyroid hormone pathway disrupted

©2015 Emily Cooper, M.D.

HOT FLASHES AND WEIGHT GAIN

A lot of women say that they didn't have weight problems until they hit menopause. But though some women do gain weight after menopause, some don't. It's not universal. Menopause can affect hormones that regulate metabolism. During menopause, estrogen which has a mainly beneficial impact on metabolism sharply declines. Since estrogen works with the hormone leptin (from fat stores) to boost metabolism, when estrogen drops, leptin may also drop, slowing metabolism in susceptible women.

And making matters worse, sleep disturbances during menopause can cause leptin levels to fall and the 'hunger hormone' ghrelin to rise—jacking up the appetite and simultaneously crashing the metabolism. Dieters are particularly susceptible to these hormone shifts because low-calorie and low-carb diets also affect leptin and ghrelin.

If you are going through menopause, keep your metabolism as healthy as possible by eating all food groups every few hours, avoid chemical food additives, get adequate sleep, and fuel exercise. Remember, cutting calories eventually lowers leptin and raises ghrelin, slowing metabolism by up to 36% within 6 months so it is almost always likely to backfire in the long run.

A HEALTHY METABOLISM:
FREE TO BURN FUEL

When the metabolism functions optimally, it stabilizes and balances the amount of energy we consume with the amount of energy we expend. We feel steady energy throughout the day. When we try to do more, our bodies provide us with more energy. Our weight consistently remains in a normal range without effort. Our brain and body maintain this balance by making often-imperceptible upward or downward adjustments that speed and slow our metabolism.

One way to think of healthy metabolic function is to compare it to driving a car. For example, say you want to drive a consistent 65 miles per hour. To stay at 65 you have to make adjustments: when you climb a hill or encounter a headwind, you press harder on the gas pedal so the car won't slow down; on the downslope, you let up on the gas or tap the brakes to slow down. Gas tank on "E"? Time to refuel.

A metabolism that operates normally is free to burn fuel at whatever rate the body requires. So when people with a healthy metabolism eat more than usual at a party or while they're on vacation, their body automatically speeds up and burns the extra fuel. If they work late and delay dinner for several hours or even skip a meal, their body taps the brakes, causing the metabolism to slow down to preserve energy until the next meal. People without weight issues don't try to control their weight by eating less or exercising more. They don't have to—their metabolism automatically balances how much energy they consume with how much they expend.

TAKING CRUISE CONTROL FOR GRANTED

Even though science tells us a healthy metabolism automatically balances fuel consumption, the story set forth in popular culture is that this balancing act requires willpower and control. According to this theory, people who don't have a weight problem or whose weight remains stable achieve this through control and willpower—by eating carefully and exercising regularly. They do everything right, which means that everyone else must be doing things wrong. When we stop to think, however, and we ignore these popular culture messages, we know this is absurd. Not only is this explanation unscientific, it's illogical.

Everyone knows somebody who eats freely or who doesn't exercise at all yet doesn't have a weight problem. Everyone also knows somebody who is careful about eating and exercise yet battles with weight—it might even be you. It's very hard to believe that a person who has never struggled with weight eats the exact same number of calories and burns that exact same number of calories every single day, day in and day out, year after year. That's what would have to happen if the conventional wisdom about the relationship between diets, exercise, and weight was hard science.

People whose metabolisms function normally may take their normal appetite and their body's weight-balancing capacity for granted. They may even wrongly believe that their diet and exercise choices are what allow their weight to remain stable. I've heard normal-weight people say more than once that if overweight people would just do everything they did, they would not have a weight problem.

WEIGHT-PRONE OR WEIGHT-RESISTANT: A MATTER OF CHANCE

Science shows us that normal-weight people are far less responsible for their weight than they may believe.

If normal-weight people are not as responsible for their weight as we have been led to believe, then logic tells us overweight people may not be responsible for theirs, either. Scientific research amassed over the past one hundred years supports this perspective; so do the cases I've witnessed firsthand in the twenty-five years I've spent treating overweight patients in my clinical practice. Weight problems most frequently develop because the metabolism is experiencing an imbalance—not because a patient is doing something wrong.

CHAPTER 7

A History of Ideas

OVER THE YEARS, THERE have been many theories about what causes obesity and overweight conditions. Some were bizarre; others made a lot of sense. Some people thought it was overeating and lack of exercise; others thought it was depression and psychological problems. Treatments for overweight have included "starvation therapy" in the early 1900s (which carried a high mortality rate), as well as medically supervised diets and exercise, which have been administered since before the 1920s. In the 1950s, theories of depression as the root cause of weight problems led to a focus on behavioral therapy, which is still popular today. Up through the present time, the medical community—and society in general—have continued to focus on diets, exercise, and behavioral treatment as the answer to obesity and overweight.

Dr. Lulu Hunt Peters, who herself struggled with weight problems, was one of the first diet advocates. In her best-selling book "Diet & Health," published in 1918, she referred to obese people as "fireless cookers" who were prone to store fat and therefore required strict caloric guidelines.

> . . . *Thin people have been proved to radiate fifty percent more heat per pound than fat people; in other words, fat people are regular fireless cookers! They hold the heat in, it cannot get out through the packing, and the food which is also contained therein goes merrily on with fiendish regularity, depositing itself as fat.*[1]

While Dr. Hunt Peters credited her health and vitality to strict adherence to her own dieting advice, she lived to only 57 years of age before succumbing to pneumonia.

---

1. Lulu Hunt Peters, Diet and Health with Key to the Calories, (Chicago: The Reilly and Lee Co., 1918): Ch. 1.

AHEAD OF THEIR TIME

Many scientific journal articles from the 1920s and '30s reveal that physicians pondered obesity in a much more analytical way than many physicians do today. One of my favorite historical accounts of the science of obesity and metabolism is from Dr. Hans Lisser's 1924 publication *The Frequency of Endogenous Endocrine Obesity and its Treatment by Glandular Therapy.*[2]

Lisser's presentation to the 53rd Annual Session of the California Medical Board and the comments in response to it show the insight of physicians of his day, in spite of their limited resources. In his presentation, Dr. Lisser explained why diet and exercise could not be considered a cure:

Radical diet restriction often reduces weight, but cannot be termed a "cure" because it fails to correct the fundamental cause of such incretory obesity . . . The chemistry of obesity is still quite obscure . . . Several glands exert a powerful influence on the shape and bulk of the human body.

2. H. Lisser, "The Frequency of Endogenous Endocrine Obesity and Its Treatment By Glandular Therapy," *Western Journal of Medicine* (October 1924), 22(10): 509–514.

Lisser pointed out that some people are clearly weight prone, and some are clearly weight resistant.

Most of us are acquainted with people who eat lightly and are very active, but who nevertheless accumulate fatty tissue. Likewise, we are aware that many persons eat heartily, are not especially athletic, and yet remain thin.

Based on his understanding of the science of his day and his observations of his own patients, Lisser concluded that diet and exercise could not "cure" the underlying cause of a weight problem, and he was eager to address the root cause rather than apply a treatment that had little chance of succeeding in the long term.

. . . Normal food intake and normal exercise will not avail with such individuals because an underlying factor is responsible which is not sufficiently recognized in diagnosis and not given proper consideration in planning treatment. This factor is an abnormal faulty metabolism, the control of which is to a large extent dominated by the glands of internal secretion.

As Lisser discusses below, even in 1924, the science—including standard endocrinology textbooks—clearly stated that hormonal issues underlie weight problems, and that excess weight is a symptom of those issues. Knowing that the theory that diets and exercise were not a cure was radical to some, Lisser carefully reminded the reader that these were not his ideas—they were established science represented in a wide range of textbooks at the time.

> *It is obviously beyond the confines of this paper to describe in detail the various types of ductless gland disease in which obesity is a common and prominent symptom . . . Many excellent textbooks are available, such as Falta, Cushing, Barker in Monographic Medicine, etc. There is nothing original in the observation that obesity is a striking symptom of incretory deficiencies.*

Many of the authors referenced here by Lisser remain famous today, including Cushing, the endocrinologist who discovered Cushing's disease.

Lisser recognized that irregular appetite is a symptom of the underlying glitches in the metabolic feedback loop. His insight in this area stemmed from research being done at the time that examined what happened in rodents when parts of the brain were cut off from communication with other parts. He didn't know that the reason for the appetite changes was specifically the impairment of MC3R activity—however, he did realize that hormones from the pituitary gland must have a role in appetite regulation, metabolic rate, and weight control.

A large appetite and a craving for sweets and starches may characterize a glutton, but it is to be remembered that this craving may itself be pathological, and depend on hypopituitarism. The hunger, thirst, and high sugar tolerance of these patients is well known. A mere restriction of food intake only scratches the surface, but neglects the underlying cause. Results would be temporary, because the patient rarely persists against an abnormal appetite difficult to control. Gland administration to supplement the patient's gland deficiency is a sound logical procedure.

In 1934, ten years after Lisser's influential paper was published, British doctor A.H. Douthwaite upheld the theory of appetite as a potential symptom rather than the cause of obesity:[3]

There is no evidence to prove that increased appetite is the primary cause of obesity. It is

3. A.H. Douthwaite, "The Treatment Of Obesity," The British Medical Journal (August 15, 1936), Vol. 2, No. 3945: 844.

conceivable that another factor, "the undeter-
minable tendency to obesity," may in itself be
responsible for the increased appetite.

Here, Dr. Douthwaite contemplates the possibilities
of a neuroendocrine cause of the problem:

In certain instances, disease of the central nervous system or dysfunction of the endocrine
glands so affects the metabolism of the body as
to favor and accelerate the generalized or local-
ized deposition of fat.

While the specific details have been better clarified in
more recent years, Drs. Lisser, Douthwaite, and their colleagues were certainly on the right track in their efforts to
outline the function of the central and peripheral metabolic pathways; in fact, their theories are still extremely
current in terms of the modern scientific view of obesity's
causes and potential treatments.

THE UNTOLD STORY

Dr. Lisser's theories about obesity were well received by
many of the endocrinology greats of the 1920s and '30s,
but the general viewpoint was still that gluttony was the

cause of weight problems. It seemed logical that individuals were gaining weight because they were eating too much. Experts did not likely understand the weight-defense system in the early 1900s, which is when some of them began encouraging diets. It was not until the 1940s and later that scientists and doctors began to realize that every type of diet they devised had a side effect: slowing of the metabolic rate.

Fortunately, scientists have made great strides in mapping out the neuroendocrine control of the metabolism, body weight, and appetite since the early 1900s. Even in 1924, scientists were already beginning to sharply challenge the "calories in, calories out" explanation of weight gain, and scientists today know that this theory is an oversimplification. We can now identify and measure many factors that not only trip the body's starvation defenses but also trigger a cascade of hormonal reactions, rendering "calories out" unpredictable and inaccurate. "Calories in, calories out" simply doesn't account for how the weight-defense system impacts the rate at which the body burns energy.

Surprisingly, in spite of the impressive body of knowledge that now exists about these topics, we still cling to a nearly one-hundred-year-old theory about why we gain weight and how to address weight problems. This is especially puzzling because the "calories in, calories out" perspective and corresponding behavioral treatments have clearly been ineffective: Americans today are actually eating less but weighing more.[4]

In the article *Obesity: Overnutrition or Disease of Metabolism?*, published in 1953 in the *American Journal of Digestive Diseases*,[5] A.W. Pennington describes his review of past studies showing that fat storage appears to be independent of energy intake:

> *Analysis of the results of studies of the energy exchange in obesity, in regard to their evidence for or against a passive dependence of the excessive energy stores on the balance between the inflow and the outflow of energy, indicates that these stores have a significant degree of independence of the energy balance.*
>
> *This appears to necessitate an explanation of obesity on the basis of some intrinsic metabolic defect.*

---

4. E.S. Ford, W.H. Dietz, "Trends in energy intake among adults in the United States: findings from NHANES," *American Journal of Clinical Nutrition* (February 20, 2013), doi: 10.3945/ajcn.112.052662.

5. A.W. Pennington, "Obesity: Overnutrition or Disease of Metabolism?," *American Journal of Digestive Diseases* (September 1953), Vol. 20, Issue 9: 268-274.

Pennington also noted that when normal-weight and overweight subjects dieted, they *both* experienced a reduction in their metabolic rate as a side effect.

> *The decline in energy expenditure which occurs when the obese go on low calorie diets appears to have the same significance as it has when people of normal weight are subjected to undernutrition.*

In his conclusion, Pennington argues that, rather than create calorie restriction (go on a diet), the solution to obesity would be to target fat stores in the body.

> *A treatment of obesity, alternate to that of caloric restriction, takes into account the metabolic defect in obesity, aims at a primary decrease in the excessive energy stores, and allows for weight reduction without any decline in the energy expenditure and without any enforcement of caloric restriction.*

Pennington was challenging the thinking of his time, but it seems he could not completely disconnect from the diet approach. He went on to experiment with liberal-calorie, low-carb diets, all of which effected only short-term success. In the process, he developed the theory that Atkins later popularized and the Paleo diet modernized. Essentially, many people today are following a diet that was first tried—without long-term success—sixty years ago.

Another article, published in the *Journal of Clinical Endocrinology and Metabolism* in 1984,[6] also found that after a diet, a patient's metabolism slowed by an amount that was proportionate to the amount of weight lost—the equivalent of 450 calories daily for someone who loses fifty pounds by dieting. This article was published thirty years after Pennington had stated that the research of his time proved this same theory: the more weight was lost, the more the metabolism slowed. E. Jéquier wrote:

After weight loss, energy expenditure decreases by about 84 kJ/24 h (20 kcal/24 h) per kg of weight loss in all patients. The need to reset energy intake to a lower level than the previous maintenance food consumption represents a major difficulty in the treatment of obesity; failure to adjust energy intake to the new requirements contributes to the frequent relapse of body weight gain in the obese after completion of a period on a hypocaloric diet.

---

6. E. Jéquier, "Energy expenditure in obesity," Journal of Clinical Endocrinology & Metabolism (November 1984): 563-580.

THE SAME OLD STORY

People often assume that as long as you exercise, your metabolism won't drop with dieting. But scientists have proven that this assumption is false. In 2012, for example, scientists performed a "biggest loser" style weight-loss diet program and measured metabolic changes. Their results confirmed past studies: after 30 weeks of dieting and intense exercise to preserve muscle mass, subjects lost 30 percent of their body weight, but their metabolisms slowed by 500 calories per day.[7]

More recent studies have examined the hormonal mechanisms behind the slowing of metabolism. An article published in the *New England Journal of Medicine* in 2011, titled "Long-term persistence of hormonal adaptations to weight loss,"[8] described a study of 50 overweight and obese patients who participated in a 10 week, very low-calorie diet. Hormone levels were measured once before the diet and twice after the diet, once at 10 weeks and once at 62 weeks. Researchers found that the diet left a lasting fingerprint on participants' levels of several hormones, including leptin and insulin, and put them in a protective mode (Diet Fog) that was likely to lead to weight regain.

7. D.L. Johannsen, N.D.Knuth, "Metabolic Slowing with Massive Weight Loss despite Preservation of Fat-Free Mass," Journal of Clinical Endocrinology & Metabolism (2012), 97(7): 2489-2496.

8. P. Sumithran, L.A. Prendergast , et al., "Long-term persistence of hormonal adaptations to weight loss," New England Journal of Medicine (October 27, 2011), 365(17), doi: 10.1056/NEJMoa1105816: 1597-1604.

> *One year after initial weight reduction, levels of*
> *the circulating mediators of appetite that encour-*
> *age weight regain after diet-induced weight loss*
> *do not revert to the levels recorded before weight*
> *loss. Long-term strategies to counteract this*
> *change may be needed to prevent obesity relapse.*

The researchers also found that patients had regained a significant amount of the weight they lost and had much higher hunger ratings.

Yet another recent study by the same researchers, published in *Clinical Science* in 2013,[9] examines the chemical changes during Diet Fog that occur as a result of dieting.

> *Diet-induced weight loss is accompanied by*
> *several physiological changes which encourage*
> *weight regain, including alterations in energy*
> *expenditure, substrate metabolism and hor-*
> *mone pathways involved in appetite regulation,*
> *many of which persist beyond the initial weight*
> *loss period.*

---

9. P. Sumithran, J. Proietto, "The defense of body weight: a physiological basis for weight regain after weight loss," Clinical Science (February 2013), 124(4), doi: 10.1042/CS20120223: 231-241.

Centuries of Discovery:

1979
The term "Impaired Glucose Tolerance" (IGT) first coined

1977
First use of the term "Metabolic Syndrome"

1973
The term "Diabesity" is coined

1960
Synthetic ACTH invented

1957
First Metformin clinical trial

1954
First reported bariatric surgery

1947
Central obesity identified as a predisposition for diabetes

1943
ACTH discovered

1936
NPH insulin invented

1935
Modern science defines type 1 & 2 diabetes

1932
First incretin discovered

1931
Insulin resistance discovered

1924
Hormonal malfunction tied to obesity

1923
Glucagon discovered

1922
Metformin synthesized

1922
Insulin given to first human subject

1921
Insulin discovered

1919
MSH discovered

1918
Calories as part of dieting introduced

1915 - 1922
Starvation diets promoted for diabetes

1902
Gut hormones first identified

1830 - 1850
BMI invented

Late 1700s
Calorimetry invented

400 - 500 AD
Type 1 & 2 diabetes understood as two conditions

1500 BCE
Diabetes described in Egyptian manuscript

Pre-1900   **Early 1900s**   **Mid 1900s**

Dieting, Hormones, Diseases & Treatments

2015
Endocrine Society releases updated
Clinical Practice Guidelines for Obesity
and recommends use of medications
to treat obesity for the first time

2014
FDA approved liraglutide
for weight loss

2014
RM-493 MC4R agonist
Phase 2 trials for obesity

2014
FDA approved combination
bupropion + naltrexone for weight loss

2013
FDA approved priority review
of Metreleptin

2012
FDA approved lorcaserin
for weight loss

2012
FDA approved combination phenterimine
+ topiramate for weight loss

2007
FTO gene associated with
obesity discovered

2006
MSH mimetic invented

2005
First GLP-1 mimetic
approved by FDA

2005
Synthetic amylin
approved by FDA

2003
Anti-ghrelin immunization
invented

2002
Synthetic oxyntomodulin
invented

2001
Synthetic PYY invented

1999
Ghrelin
discovered

1999
First human trials
using Metreleptin

1998
FDA approved
glucagon injection

1996
Adiponectin
discovered

1995
Metformin
released in the U.S.

1994
Leptin
discovered

1987
Amylin
discovered

1982
Oxyntomodulin
discovered

1982
Neuropeptide Y
(NPY) discovered

1980
PYY discovered

The future

Late 1900s   **Early 2000s**

Over the decades, researchers have proven time and time again that dieting is a short-term strategy that triggers the body's weight defenses. The body can detect deprivation—you can't trick it into losing weight long term by reducing your calorie intake—so dieting has little chance of solving weight problems in the long run.

Even before Pennington's time, hundreds of studies showed the same results. Information about diets not working in the long term and about diets slowing the metabolism is now included as established fact in every textbook on obesity or metabolism. So why hasn't public opinion changed?

CHALLENGING OUR ASSUMPTIONS

Recent research has expanded the scientific investigation of weight problems to associations other than dieting and exercise. For example, a study examining snacking in teens shows that teens who snacked were not at increased risk of obesity, and in fact some studies show that teens who snack are at a lower risk for obesity, even when their snacks are fast-food based.[10]

10. N. Larson, et al., "A review of snacking patterns among children and adolescents: what are the implications of snacking for weight status," Child Obesity Journal (April 2013), 9(2) doi: 10.1089/chi.2012.0108: 104-115.

One study examined the association between sleep and teens with a propensity for overweight: it found that teens who slept more than 7.5 hours per night showed a lower risk for obesity.[11] Another study revealed that nearly 7,000 kids who participated in an intensive physical activity program in school exhibited no association between their activity and their body weight or body fat levels.[12] Still other studies have shown that "food deserts"— places where there is a lack of fresh food and increased availability of fast food—are actually not associated with an increased risk of overweight and obesity.[13]

In the face of the repeated long-term failures of diets, many researchers are still talking about trying to figure out how to trick the body into not sensing deprivation during deprivation diets. But based on almost one hundred years of existing research, and the success I've witnessed with my patients, I'm convinced that the better approach is to apply the science of metabolism and avoid diets altogether. Why diet or try to trick our bodies when we can potentially detect and correct the true underlying causes of overweight and obesity, rendering those other measures unnecessary?

11. J.A. Mitchell, D. Rodriguez, et al., "Sleep Duration and Adolescent Obesity," Pediatrics (April 8, 2013), doi: 10.1542/peds: 2012-2368.

12. J. Deardorff, "Measuring body fat may weigh on students' self-image," Chicago Tribune, June 9, 2013.

13. D. Viola, P.S. Arno, A.R. Maroko, et al., "Overweight and obesity: Can we reconcile evidence about supermarkets and fast food retailers for public health policy?," Journal of Public Health Policy (May 30, 2013), doi: 10.1057/jphp.2013.19.

CHAPTER 8

Weight Loss Resistance: A Veritable Firewall

WEIGHT PROBLEMS OCCUR for many reasons, but most have genetic roots—in fact, scientists believe that up to 70 percent of obesity is genetically based. A combination of genetic and environmental factors creates glitches in the metabolic feedback loop, causing the body and brain to inaccurately perceive starvation. Potential triggers of this malfunction include:

- undiagnosed and undertreated gestational diabetes
- puberty hormones

- medications (certain antidepressants or psychotropic medications, birth control, steroids like prednisone and cortisone shots, most sleep medications, and certain cholesterol and blood pressure medications)
- environmental toxins (found in cosmetics, plastics, fragrances, pollution, pesticides, etc.)
- sleep deprivation or sleep apnea
- dieting or under-fueled exercise

WHAT'S TRIGGERING THE EPIDEMIC?

In spite of the input from a multitude of science reports, all we ever hear is that people are eating too much and not moving enough. And the media constantly depicts people with obesity eating french fries while those with normal weight are eating light yogurt and exercising. And that is simply not the case in real life. I see many patients with high body weight who are exercising more and eating less when they first come to see me than my normal weight patients are. I'm frequently asked if it's not too much food and not enough exercise, what's triggering the epidemic?

There are many other factors, and contrary to popular thinking they are usually not within a person's control

What's triggering this epidemic?

GENETIC VULNERABILITY

Lifestyle
- Dieting • Restrictive Mindset
- Underfueled Exercise
- Stress • Skimping on Sleep

Sleep
- Lack of Quality Sleep
- Sleep Apnea

Gestational Diabetes
- Underdiagnosed • Undertreated

Environmental Obesogens
- BPA • Food Additives • Pesticides
- Phthalates • Secondhand Smoke

Medications
- SSRIs • Benzodiazepines • Steroids
- Atypical Anti-psychotics • Birth Control
- Many Sleep Meds • Some Pain Meds
- Some BP / Cholesterol Meds
- Maternal Fertility Treatments

Food Insecurity
- Poverty

METABOLIC DYSFUNCTION

Hypoglycemia

Infertility

Type 2 Diabetes

Obesity

Cardiovascular Risk
High Blood Pressure
High Cholesterol

©2015 Emily Cooper, M.D.

with just lifestyle strategies alone. Especially if you have a family history of obesity or diabetes you may be particularly vulnerable to several potential triggers.

Dieting causes biological adaptation, the body's way of protecting itself from perceived starvation. Irregular eating, skipping meals, omitting food groups and under-fueled exercise can also contribute. Not getting enough sleep, sleep apnea, and even certain widely used medications can promote obesity. And many common chemicals have been identified as potential obesogens, including artificial sweeteners, emulsifiers, plastic packaging and even synthetic carpeting.

People living in poverty may not have access to a consistent food supply. This is why simply changing the quality of food available in a low income neighborhood doesn't equate to a reduction in obesity rates. Without access to food on a consistent basis, the body tends to hold on to extra fat for protection.

And because gestational diabetes is often underdiagnosed and undertreated in our country, obesity and diabetes risk in both mother and child is accelerated.

Yet we still constantly hear that sugar is the culprit that correlates with obesity, and this is professed across the country, but many other factors, such as the increasing rate of plastic production in the U.S., coincide with the simultaneous increase in obesity.

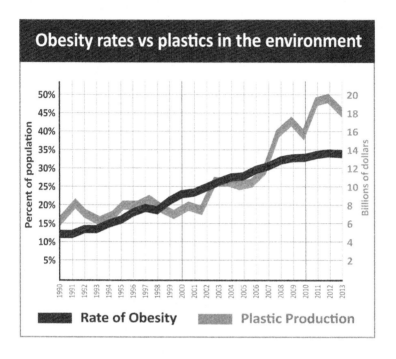

It's also a fact that as we cut cut down on cigarette smoking the obesity rates increased. What is interesting is that nicotine reduces starvation signals in the brain, in particular neuropeptide Y, a starvation neurotransmitter that plays a major role in appetite and energy expenditure. So the true obesity rates may have been masked while our country was tied up with cigarette smoking. Of course smoking is detrimental to our health so that's clearly not the answer! But certain medications used in the treatment of obesity actually create a similar physiologic effect on metabolism without the harmful effects of smoking.

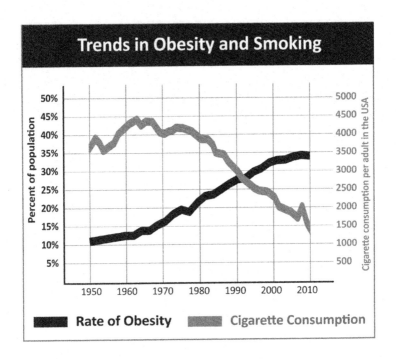

METABOLIC STORM

When glitches in our metabolic feedback loop cause the body to perceive that we are starving, it acts defensively, simultaneously lowering our metabolic rate and compelling us to consume more fuel. If we ignore this drive to eat, our body simply slows our metabolism even further in an attempt to meet its protective goal of defending or increasing its fat mass. I refer to the powerful malfunctions of the metabolic feedback loop that promote and protect excess body weight as the "Metabolic Storm".

There are numerous common warning signs of an

underlying hormonal imbalance, and they differ among people—in fact, a person can experience different warning signs at different times throughout their life. These include:

- constant hunger
- not feeling satisfied after eating
- frequent and sudden feelings of an overly full stomach
- a preoccupation with food
- indecision about whether to eat and what to eat
- cravings for sweets or high-fat foods
- low energy
- reproductive system and growth issues in both males and females (irregular periods, abnormal testosterone, infertility, precocious puberty in girls, slowing of height increase in adolescents)

THESE GLITCHES ARE BITCHES

Short circuits in the metabolic feedback loop activate a series of defenses that adjust the behavior of not just one hormone or body system, but *several* of them—and all at once. These adjustments form a veritable firewall against body fat loss and, ultimately, starvation. The brain and body may have activated the weight-defense system based on an inaccurate perception of the situation, but their goal is no different than it would be were they experiencing actual starvation: to defend body mass by causing metabolic slowdown and weight gain.

There are numerous hormonal glitches that can cause disproportionate weight gain or weight-loss resistance, including insulin resistance, adiponectin deficiency, low leptin, leptin resistance, incretin deficiency, amylin malfunction, and ghrelin excess. As you will discover, all of these malfunctions can result in elevated blood sugar, insulin imbalance, slowing metabolism, weight gain, and appetite deregulation. We'll begin with insulin resistance.

Insulin Resistance

You may remember that insulin helps bring glucose and proteins into the body tissues so they can utilize them for energy. By removing glucose from the blood and carrying it into the tissues, insulin helps keep blood glucose from getting too high. Insulin also reassures the brain that we are nourished. One of the many ways in which the body accumulates fat is through a medical problem called *insulin resistance*.

Insulin resistance is characterized by a lack of response by the muscle tissue and often the brain to the effects of insulin. This resistance makes it more difficult for glucose to enter the cells—potentially leading to an increase in circulating blood glucose and insulin levels, telling the body to store rather than burn fat. This is a very common problem among people who are overweight or obese. Since insulin is an anabolic hormone, elevated levels lead to increasing body mass, both fat and lean mass. And although muscle tissue can become resistant to insulin, limiting its ability to store glucose, fat mass does not become insensitive to insulin, so as insulin levels rise, energy floods into the fat stores easily. Luckily, insulin resistance is reversible—but if left untreated, the pancreas's insulin-producing cells can eventually fatigue, increasing the risk of glucose buildup in the blood. At this point, insulin resistance progresses to pre-diabetes and then type 2 diabetes, which is why I often call insulin resistance "pre-pre-diabetes."

Insulin resistance can exist as part of *metabolic syndrome*, the diagnosis criteria being a minimum of three of the following features:

- elevated glucose or insulin levels
- cholesterol abnormalities (elevated triglycerides, elevated LDL particles, and/or low HDL)
- elevated blood pressure
- increased waist circumference

In women, insulin resistance can also be associated with a condition called *polycystic ovarian syndrome* (PCOS). PCOS is characterized by irregular menses, increased facial hair growth, acne, and infertility. There are lab tests that can detect PCOS, and a pelvic ultrasound can sometimes reveal numerous tiny ovarian cysts.

In men, insulin resistance can contribute to low testosterone and sometimes excess estrogen. Symptoms of these hormonal imbalances in men include increased belly fat, increased breast tissue, low energy and motivation, poor concentration, and low sex drive.

Scientists have found that insulin resistance may develop as a result of deeper underlying malfunctions. One of these potential triggers can be an adiponectin deficiency. As you may recall, adiponectin is an insulin sensitizer, so when it declines, muscle insulin sensitivity also can decline, causing insulin resistance. For other patients, inappropriately high insulin spikes after meals can cause dramatic drops in blood sugar. When this happens repeatedly, the body may eventually become resistant to the excessive circulating insulin to defend itself against low-blood-sugar reactions.

A common symptom of insulin resistance can be sugar cravings, because the muscles feel starved of glucose. A fairly frequent physical sign of the disorder is *acanthosis nigricans*, a condition characterized by a darkening and thickening of skin in the folds of the body and on the knuckles. Stretch marks can also occur in people suffering from insulin resistance, particularly darker-skinned people.

Research has shown that weight gain is often a symptom—not a cause—of insulin resistance. In insulin resistance, high insulin turns the body's fat-burning switch off and the fat-storing switch on. As belly fat increases, however, it contributes to the problem by releasing specialized hormones that exacerbate insulin resistance and promote even more fat gain. This vicious cycle is a good example of how metabolic hormones communicate with and support each other, in a sometimes misguided attempt to ensure the body's survival.

As excess insulin makes blood vessels stiffer and thicker, the passageway through them narrows, a condition called *hypertrophy*. Hypertrophy increases blood pressure and can cause small blood vessels to close up, leading to heart attack or stroke.

People with a family history of diabetes, with a personal history of insulin resistance, pre-diabetes or gestational diabetes, or who were born to a mother who had gestational diabetes, are at a higher risk of developing diabetes. However, not everyone with insulin resistance is destined to develop diabetes—especially if they take steps to treat their condition.

Break A World Record,
Win Olympic Medals—
But "Put the Waffle Down, Margaret!"

Margaret[1] dreamed of becoming an Olympic swimmer from a young age—and she eventually reached that goal, participating in two Olympic Games. In 2008, while competing in her second Olympic Games in Beijing, Margaret won two silver medals and one bronze medal. At one point in her career she even held a world record in the 200-meter backstroke.

As early as age eleven, however, and throughout her swimming career, no matter how hard Margaret trained, she struggled with her weight. "Even being as fit as I was, my coaches were never happy with my weight," she recalled.

With trainers pushing her to improve her body composition, Margaret restricted the types of foods she ate and cut both her calorie and her carb intake for years. She always felt tired, and she noticed that it took her longer to recover from workouts than it did her teammates. Even at the top of her game—even while holding a world record—her coaches basically told her to "put the waffle down." She was the fastest swimmer in the world in her signature event, the 200-meter backstroke, and yet she still wasn't good enough.

"I knew that my body was different when I compared myself to my college roommates. I watched how they ate. I ate no differently than they did, but I was bigger. It was

1. Margaret Hoelzer gave permission to use her real name in this book.

more difficult for my weight to balance in a range normally attributed to highly competitive swimmers," Margaret said. The fact that she didn't "fit the profile" physically was very distressing to her, as her coaches continually focused on cutting back her food and her rest.

Finally, Margaret decided that she had had enough. Tired of feeling run down and hungry, she retired. As soon as she stopped her heavy Olympic-level training, however, Margaret gained weight rapidly. That's when she came to see me.

Like most patients struggling with weight, I discovered that Margaret had an underlying medical problem: insulin resistance. This condition, in addition to the strict diet and intense exercise regimen she had adhered to for many years, was causing her body to fiercely defend her weight. Although even Olympic athletes are rarely screened for them, the types of problems Margaret was experiencing are actually very common.

Like many other patients who struggle with their weight, Margaret burst into tears when I explained that her weight problems weren't her fault. "My entire life I'd been told that it was something I was doing wrong," she cried.

Not true. And imagine what such an accomplished champion could have achieved if she had not been battling a metabolic problem the entire time she was competing, and hadn't been starved and tired to boot.

The fact that insulin resistance causes the body to store fat is one of the most important reasons we have far less control over our weight than popular culture purports. People with insulin resistance can eat the same foods in the same quantities as people without the condition, but their body stores more fat in response, making it virtually impossible for them to lose weight.

Adiponectin Deficiency

In a normally functioning metabolism, fat emits adiponectin to inform the rest of the body about how much fat it's carrying. Adiponectin helps lean mass become more sensitive to insulin, allowing glucose to enter the tissue cells more easily. Adiponectin also increases metabolic rate and reduces inflammation throughout the body and within blood vessels.

But sometimes adiponectin levels drop. Scientists have observed that this malfunction can occur suddenly, as though something pulled a "trigger" metabolically. Many medications and environmental toxins common to our daily life have been implicated as possible culprits. Researchers believe that people with a genetic predisposition for diabetes are more vulnerable to "obesogens," which are environmental chemicals that disrupt the endocrine system, altering adiponectin and other metabolic hormone levels.

Obesogens include common household toxins like

bisphenol A (BPA), phthalates, and food additives like emulsifiers and even artificial sweeteners.

A recent study showed that teen girls who tested as having the highest BPA levels also had the highest BMIs.[2] Similar to many earlier studies, this showed a direct correlation between environmental toxins and metabolic issues. Metabolic disruption has also been traced to the womb, so there is no way to know if a suppression of adiponectin has occurred prenatally.

Some of my patients can identify a specific time in their life when their body weight became difficult to control, and it's often tied to when they started taking a particular medication. Most sleep medications—antianxiety, antipsychotic, and antidepressant medications; certain cholesterol and blood pressure medications; certain pain medications; prednisone and cortisone shots; and some forms of birth control or progesterone—can cause metabolic disruptions, including adiponectin suppression. Interestingly, sixty percent of my new patients with obesity report having taken a steroid medication, like prednisone or cortisone, in the past.

In addition to promoting insulin resistance, an adiponectin deficiency can also reduce the body's metabolic burn rate, both at rest and during exercise. In fact, many studies have shown that overweight children and adults

2. C. Petrochko, "BPA Level Tied to Higher Weight in Girls," MedPage Today (June 12, 2013).

frequently burn less fuel when they're resting and exercising than do normal-weight people.

Low Leptin

Fat cells emit leptin to inform the brain and body of body mass and fat status. With normal metabolic function, leptin levels represent body mass accurately, and we feel satisfied after eating. The body burns glucose normally and doesn't store excess fat. Normal body weight is maintained automatically with no added effort. But dieting (which is the most common cause of leptin suppression), under-fueled exercise, or low-blood-sugar reactions can suppress leptin levels disproportionate to the amount of body mass. In dieting, for example, fat begins to emit abnormally low amounts of leptin; in essence, the fat mass is hiding by emitting less leptin, blinding the brain from seeing the fat stores and making it believe the body weighs much less than it actually does.

This state, also called *hypoleptinemia* or *acquired leptin insufficiency*, is triggered by and accentuates the body's weight-defense response. The brain and body shift into energy-conservation mode, storing fat. This is what is happening during the diet plateau and subsequent regain period. Once leptin drops very low, the metabolism slows and excess hunger may become a biological response. Weight gain, then, is not the result of going off a diet—biology actually stops the weight loss and starts the weight gain *before* a diet ends. From the brain and body's distorted perspective, the body is not merely un-dernourished—it no longer carries enough fat tissue to ensure survival.

Leptin levels can drop unnaturally low in as little as 72 hours after a person starts dieting. These hormonal changes that trigger the weight-defense system in response to restrictive eating—what I refer to as "Diet Fog"—are the underlying cause of the short-lived success of diets.

Scientists have repeatedly found that after a 12-week diet and exercise program, leptin levels often remain sup-pressed for a minimum of one to two years and it is not clear whether they ever naturally return to baseline pre-diet levels. Leptin can also drop due to inadequate sleep. Cutting back on food intake to squeeze into a wedding dress, participating in a "detox," or trying to make weight for a sports event can push the body beyond its tipping point and into self-preservation mode.

Leptin Resistance

Leptin resistance causes the brain and body to wrongly be-lieve that the body isn't carrying sufficient fat for survival, in spite of normal or elevated leptin levels in circulation. This triggers the body's weight defense system—shutting down metabolism, increasing the appetite, reducing satiety, and causing the body to conserve energy and store more fat.

In my practice, I often see leptin resistance in patients following a period of dieting, a few months after the diet is over. Leptin levels can drop dramatically during a diet—disproportionate to the amount of weight lost. After dropping, it may eventually sharply rebound to an abnormally high level, or to a normal level, but with impaired signaling in the brain. Increased ghrelin or decreased amylin (both known side effects of dieting) can be the cause of this impaired signaling—ghrelin by blocking leptin's signals, and amylin by failing to help the brain see the leptin. Leptin resistance can also be aggravated by sleep apnea, which impairs both leptin and ghrelin levels.

Some of the most important receptor sites that can become resistant to leptin signals reside in the brain, liver, and pancreas. These sites significantly impact weight, glucose, and insulin regulation. The metabolic pathway breaks down when the brain is resistant to leptin signals—the appetite receptors don't receive signals that the body has sufficient mass, and the metabolism slows, resulting in the symptoms I've described before: an increased urge to forage, constant hunger, and a lack of satiety after eating.

This metabolic backlash is characterized by an acceleration of weight regain to at least the point of the pre-diet weight, and frequently beyond it—and once this process is initiated, it's difficult to bring it under control.

Incretin Deficiency

Another way the metabolism can fool the brain into thinking it's starving and it should preserve and store body fat is by turning down or turning off incretins like GLP-1. This *incretin malfunction* occurs in dieting, anorexia, pre-diabetes, and diabetes. Deficient incretin levels cause miscommunication in the metabolic feedback loop: the brain doesn't receive the signal confirming fuel has been consumed. When this occurs, people often continue to feel hungry and unsatisfied after a normal-sized meal, and the metabolism slows.

With deficient GLP-1, in addition to the brain not acknowledging consumed fuel, the stomach empties faster and the gut takes the brakes off the pace at which glucose and other nutrients pass into the bloodstream, causing blood glucose levels to elevate. As a result, the body stores more glucose than normal as fat.

Amylin Malfunction

People with metabolic problems can frequently be either *amylin resistant* or *amylin deficient*. Amylin is secreted from the pancreas with insulin, so when insulin output is high, amylin output is as well. When hormone levels become too high, receptors lose their sensitivity to amylin and become resistant to its effects. On the other hand, people who diet or have anorexia may instead experience *suppressed* insulin and amylin output, causing them to be *amylin deficient*. In either case, there are similar metabolic consequences.

Amylin's major functions are to make the brain see the leptin signal more clearly and to regulate the pace of stomach emptying, nutrient absorption, and glucagon secretion from the pancreas. Amylin-signaling problems can cause: the brain to remain resistant to leptin even when leptin levels are normal; rapid stomach emptying that pours a flood of nutrients into the bloodstream, triggering excess insulin output; and excessive glucagon secretion, triggering glucose dumping from the liver into the bloodstream.

Ghrelin Excess

Ghrelin is secreted by the stomach. In normal conditions, ghrelin increases during fasting and before meals. *Ghrelin excess* is usually triggered by dieting or anorexia, though sleep deprivation and sleep apnea can also contribute. With ghrelin excess, baseline ghrelin levels elevate above normal and do not decline after eating, which means that although the body has been fueled, ghrelin continues to signal to the brain that there is a need for food.

People often refer to ghrelin as the "hunger hormone," but my patients with high ghrelin levels don't necessarily report feeling excessively hungry. The primary symptom that patients report is persistent, steady, and sometimes rapid weight gain, and weight-loss resistance in spite of all their efforts. In combination with decreased leptin and amylin, increased ghrelin usually precipitates weight-regain backlash after a diet—and it can get "stuck" in an elevated position, contributing to long-term weight-loss resistance.

A 'MULTI-METABOLIC HORMONAL DISEASE STATE'

As you learned in Chapter 1 many medical organizations describe the multitude of potential glitches in the metabolic feedback loop as a multi-metabolic hormonal disease state. In reality, many patients have numerous imbalances because one glitch can lead to another. Sometimes these glitches affect areas we never associate with metabolism, like fertility. In fact, numerous metabolic hormones and neurotransmitters can disturb reproduc-

When metabolic dysfunction is the root cause and excess weight is a symptom...

Obesity

Type 2 Diabetes

Cardiovascular Risk
High Blood Pressure
High Cholesterol

METABOLIC DYSFUNCTION

Hypoglycemia

Infertility

©2015 Emily Cooper, M.D.

tive function in both men and women, limiting fertility and potentially increasing pregnancy complications. Excess insulin, ghrelin, AgRP or NPY and/or deficient leptin and MSH can inhibit fertility in both men and women.

Another interesting and destructive form of metabolic malfunction involves crashing blood sugar (glucose) levels after eating: i.e., hypoglycemia. Normally, after eating, blood sugar levels increase; however, in some people they actually do the opposite. When blood sugar levels drop after eating, it's confusing to the brain and can interrupt normal signals traveling through the metabolic feedback loop. This can become a vicious cycle because the disrupted feedback loop provokes even more blood sugar crashes after eating. In addition to being an enormous contributor to abnormal weight gain, hypoglycemia causes symptoms like sleepiness, anxiety, irritability, and headaches. This situation can also provoke pre-diabetes because the body tries desperately to compensate for hypoglycemia (after meals) by raising fasting glucose levels.

DIET FOG: ONE THING ON TOP OF ANOTHER

Once an underlying hormonal imbalance develops, whether in early childhood or not until adulthood, people often find themselves between a rock and a hard place. If they diet, they temporarily lose weight, but regardless of how much they shed, the weight always seems to eventually return.

When a person with metabolic pathway glitches goes on a diet, Diet Fog always sets in at some point, creating a secondary problem that amplifies the underlying Metabolic Storm.

Symptoms of Diet Fog are:

- plateau in weight loss
- weight gain
- fatigue
- intense fear of weight regain

Once the body sees the diet as deprivation, a starvation response kicks into gear—the brain and body essentially dial 911, mobilizing resources in order to survive. Scientific research has shown that a person's metabolism can slow by 400 to 500 calories a day within weeks of beginning a diet and up to 36% within six months of starting the diet. You may wonder how this slowing occurs. Research shows leptin levels fall 65% and ghrelin levels rise 45% immediately after an eight-week diet, and they remain off balance for years after just that one diet. This helps to explain why most dieters plateau and then eventually gain back the weight that they lost (and often even more than that)—five hundred calories is what many people cut out of their daily intake when they diet, so when their metabolism slows that much, they're barely breaking even.

Just as you might turn down your thermostat and unplug appliances to reduce your carbon footprint or save money on home utility bills, the brain and body have their own ways of saving energy. The metabolism can reduce the flow of nutrients to non-essential body functions—slowing

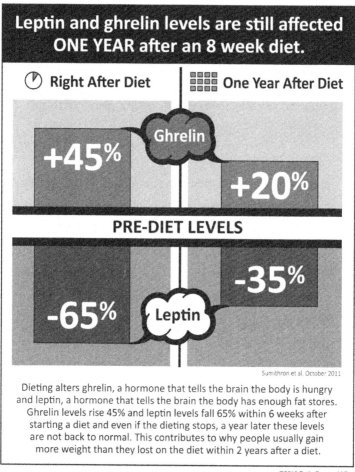

Leptin and ghrelin levels are still affected ONE YEAR after an 8 week diet.

Right After Diet   One Year After Diet

Ghrelin

+45%

+20%

PRE-DIET LEVELS

-35%

-65%   Leptin

Sumithron et al. October 2011

Dieting alters ghrelin, a hormone that tells the brain the body is hungry and leptin, a hormone that tells the brain the body has enough fat stores. Ghrelin levels rise 45% and leptin levels fall 65% within 6 weeks after starting a diet and even if the dieting stops, a year later these levels are not back to normal. This contributes to why people usually gain more weight than they lost on the diet within 2 years after a diet.

down hair and nail growth, decreasing body temperature a fraction of a degree, or apportioning less fuel for immediate use, causing energy levels to decline. Also, because compared to survival, childbearing is a "want" and not a "must," both men and women can become less fertile. The brain

JUST THE FACTS

Scientific evidence shows that diet, exercise, and other lifestyle changes do not permanently correct hormone imbalances or the weight gain that these imbalances cause.

and body may also decide to repair fewer cells, which may cause the body to ache or sustain injury more easily, or to redirect incoming fuel to pad the body's fat-storage areas.

Remember Kate, the Ironman competitor who couldn't understand why she gained sixty-five pounds when she was eating carefully and exercising fifteen to twenty hours per week? It turns out that Kate had metabolic syndrome that caused her to store fat from an early age. It's a very common condition—in fact, nearly 40 percent of U.S. adults in her demographic group suffer from metabolic syndrome—and it is potentially reversible with treatment. There is little scientific evidence, however, that dieting and exercise can "cure" this problem long term. Rather, recent studies show that this syndrome can actually become more intense after dieting, just as Kate's weight came back in spite of a low caloric intake and high exercise expenditure. Her extreme calorie deficit only exacerbated her body's fear of deprivation and amplified its weight-storing system, adding gasoline to the fire.

Once the weight-defense system has been triggered, nothing—no diet, no eating plan, no "superfood," and no exercise regimen—can outsmart the disaster drills, backup plans, and fail-safes orchestrated by the brain and body.

DNA: GETTING TO THE ROOT OF THE PROBLEM

The propensity for metabolic malfunction exists in most of us, at least in one way or another. In those of us with prominent genetic vulnerabilities—people who are weight prone rather than weight resistant—it doesn't take much to disrupt our metabolism.

You can't really identify the precise root causes of metabolic malfunction without looking at DNA code. Research has shown that DNA affects insulin and leptin receptors, as well as factors like how much insulin, leptin, and POMC the body produces, and how sensitive the leptin receptors, MC3Rs, and MC4Rs are. To date, scientists have identified nearly one hundred genetic variations and hundreds of specific genetic mutations that can contribute to weight-prone tendencies.[3] For example, some people may lack an enzyme required to prevent

3. B.M. Herrera, S. Keildson, C.M. Lindgren, "Genetics and epigenetics of obesity," Maturitas (May 2011), 69(1) doi: 10.1016/j.maturitas.2011.02.018 PMCID: PMC3213306: 41–49.

MSH from being too sticky. When MSH is too sticky, it glues itself to other molecules and becomes too bulky to fit easily into the "lock" that opens the MC4Rs (Door Four). Another variation may cause MSH to pick up an incorrect amino acid, changing its shape and preventing it from fitting into the receptors correctly. Some people experience other genetic vulnerabilities that slow down the pace of the communication pathway in their brain. And when *epigenetic changes* occur—when a person's original genes get modified over time—a pre-existing genetic tendency can surface or intensify. In theory, these genetic conditions can alter the brain receptors, making it more difficult for them to pick up hormonal signals.

Genetic variants affecting the metabolic feedback loop make some people more vulnerable to weight problems than others. When we compare the same locations on the DNA strands of people with and without weight problems, in fact, we often find that those without weight problems have built-in weight resistance. This might be because they have more than the normal amount of receptors, because their receptors are more sensitive to the signals, or because their receptors are resistant to shutting down. Regardless, the end result is the same: they are more resistant to factors that can contribute to weight gain.

THANKS, MOM AND DAD

Many people experience weight challenges associated with their genetics. For example, a family history of type 2 diabetes or obesity is highly associated with a vulnerability to weight problems. In addition to genetic influences, children born at a low birth weight, children who went hungry in early life, children or adolescents who engaged in dieting at an early age, and those exposed to high levels of environmental obesogens are more vulnerable to adult overweight and obesity. This is also true for babies born to a mother with gestational diabetes. Babies born between 1940 and 1970 to women taking the drug DES (diethylstilbestrol) during pregnancy can also have an increased risk of future weight problems and increased diabetes risk. Tests from umbilical cord blood at birth show that alterations in the fat cell hormones leptin and adiponectin are associated with greater risk of overweight and obesity in the offspring by as early as age three to six years old.[4]

When nine-year-old Olivia came to see me, her body weight was already in a range that's considered extremely high, even for adults, and she reported an abnormally elevated appetite and significant fatigue. The tests I ran showed that, due to her genetics and to unknown triggers

4. C.S. Mantzoros, S.L. Rifas-Shiman, et al., "Cord Blood Leptin and Adiponectin as Predictors of Adiposity in Children at 3 Years of Age: A Prospective Cohort Study," Pediatrics (February 2009), 123(2), doi: 10.1542/peds.2008-0343, PMCID: PMC2761663: 682–689.

174 THE METABOLIC STORM

(which were most probably encountered in the womb), Olivia had a severe case of insulin and leptin resistance. She had a number of glitches in her metabolic feedback loop.

It was difficult to manage Olivia's metabolic malfunctions because she was a child, and because, as in many cases of pediatric obesity and insulin resistance, her metabolic malfunctions were very strong. There are few medications that can be used by patients so young. Because of this, it was extremely difficult to medically treat Olivia and make an impact on correcting her metabolism, especially in the first few years I treated her. It was even more important than usual for her to get to bed on time and eat balanced meals and snacks, and the last thing a child or pre-teen wants to think about is healthy habits—taking medications, eating balanced meals, going to bed on time, and seeing doctors regularly. Her parents had to monitor her medication and supplement regimen to ensure she was on track. Her dad also took the time to join Olivia in physical activities she enjoyed, such as swimming, to help with her mobility.

In time, Olivia's health improved—and now, after years of work and in spite of the severity of her metabolic problem, we have finally begun to break through her powerful weight defenses. Her weight gain has not only stopped, it has begun a consistent downward trajectory. No amount of dieting and exercise could have fixed Olivia's Metabolic

Storm. Her issues had to be addressed with a comprehensive program that included a regular schedule of supplements and targeted medication suitable for an adolescent.

FEAST OR FAMINE

A popular theory about what makes some of us more weight prone than others is that some of us have remote or recent ancestors who experienced more famine than others. Although many people living in today's developed world give little thought to famines, they are among the oldest and most dangerous risks known to humankind. Where threats to our wellbeing are concerned, they rank up there with perils like lacking access to shelter and water, drowning, and being attacked by predators.

Although many of us use the phrase "dying from hunger" as a figure of speech, many of our forebears literally lived from feast to famine. The DNA of those who survived became encoded with data about how to endure food shortages. Our genes carry this knowledge forward from generation to generation, some experts believe. This survival mechanism protects us. It is so powerful that the brain and body of modern-day humans automatically assume that they are in danger unless hormonal signals convince them that the body is nutritionally safe and has an adequate, secure food supply and sufficient fat mass.

By studying the great famines throughout history, scientists have found that people whose ancestors survived famine conditions have a higher risk of developing weight problems than the descendants of ancestors whose food supply was never in peril. Gillian, whose ancestors were Irish farmers, is an excellent example of this. Obesity runs throughout her family tree, and when she was just a child, her concerned parents sent her to a diet clinic so she "wouldn't turn out like her obese relatives."

"I started dieting in second grade," Gillian reported. Her weight began to increase at an early age and continued to rise into adulthood, although she ate healthfully and stayed active. Eventually, at 400 pounds, Gillian resorted to gastric bypass surgery. "But now," she said, "I've regained almost of the weight I lost since my surgery ten years ago."

Like many other people who struggle with weight problems, Gillian has a genetic vulnerability to obesity—her body's weight-defense system, strongly influenced by her DNA, causes glitches in her metabolic feedback loop, and her past dieting and surgery have only amplified those glitches. No matter which tactic she uses, if she tries to lose weight her brain perceives it as deprivation, and it tells her body to store everything as fat for protection. Now, however, by identifying and treating her specific underlying glitches—which include metabolic syndrome and leptin resistance—she is finally beginning to address the problem at its root. This process will not take place overnight; it took years for Gillian to get to the point where she is now, and it will take even more time for her metabolism to shift to a less weight-defensive mode. But we are encouraged by the positive changes that are already beginning to take place in her health and weight trends.

WHAT CAN WE DO?

Research of the past two decades suggests that medically realigning the metabolic feedback loop is the key to long-term results when it comes to dealing with weight issues. It has also shown that hormonal irregularities that cause overweight and obesity cannot be corrected through any amount of willpower or control; these irregularities are caused by physiological problems, not behavior problems, and therefore they can only be solved through medical treatment. There are medications available today that can help most people correct metabolic malfunctions—and the more advancements we make in this area, the closer we are to revolutionizing the way society as a whole deals with weight problems. When it comes to overweight and obesity, science holds the answers.

CHAPTER 9

What Does the Metabolic System Have to Do With Fertility? Everything!

According to the CDC, there are nearly 7 million women with impaired fertility in America. Estimates are that about 12% of men and women in the U.S. have problems with infertility.[1] We always hear about infertility and fertility treatment so it's surprising that levels of infertility have plateaued over the past decade and even have decreased slightly.

---

1. Chandra A, Copen CE, Stephen EH. Infertility and impaired fecundity in the United States, 1982–2010: Data from the National Survey of Family Growth. National health statistics reports; no 67. Hyattsville, MD: National Center for Health Statistics. 2013

Men's metabolic function can affect their testosterone levels—sex drive, sexual function, and sperm characteristics. Therefore, for men, glitches in the metabolic pathway can affect all of these areas. In general, pituitary gland hormones regulate testosterone and sperm production, and what's interesting is that male sperm counts and testosterone levels are on the decline in North America.[2] And some reports suggest that men today would never qualify as sperm donors using the standards of twenty years ago. There are many possible factors that can contribute to this drop, including environmental endocrine-disrupting chemicals that we are exposed to on a daily basis (phthalates, BpA, plasticizers).

Like their male counterparts, women's fertility is also greatly impacted by factors linked to metabolism. Yet when women seek medical attention for infertility, they usually don't undergo an intensive workup to identify the cause. The main goal in reproductive medicine immediately shifts towards stimulating pregnancy in most cases, rather than diagnosis or treatment of the infertility itself. Therefore, it's not surprising that root causes of a woman's infertility are often missed.

Reproduction is critically dependent on metabolism.[3] In order to understand the connection, you will need an

2. Travison TG, AB Araujo, AB O'Donnell, et al., "A Population-level Decline in Serum Testosterone Levels in American Men," Journal of Clinical Endocrinology and Metabolism (2007), Vol. 92 No. 1: 196-202, doi: 10.1210/jc.2006-1375

3. Michalakis K, G Mintziori, A Kaprara, et al., "The Complex Interaction Between Obesity, Metabolic Syndrome and Reproductive Axis: A Narrative Review," Metabolism (2013), Vol. 62 No. 4: 457-478

introduction to reproductive endocrinology! It may sound complicated but it's really mostly common sense. There's a sequence of events that is coordinated from the higher levels of the brain to the reproductive organs. The incoming signals from the peripheral system to the brain, which indicate the body is nutritionally safe, are critical for having a healthy reproductive pathway. After all, why would the body allow you to reproduce if it perceives that your own body is in danger nutritionally? So let's delve into the body's process related to fertility and explain this connection.

The testicles in men and the ovaries in women are called *gonads*. They are responsible for generating sex hormones (testosterone and estrogen) and for various aspects of reproduction. Both testicular and ovarian function are actually directed by the brain, and not the thinking brain, but the chemical signals produced by the brain. These signals that the brain generates are greatly influenced by the the peripheral metabolic pathway, and many of the same signals we spoke of that regulate weight, appetite, and energy expenditure. In addition to the players we've already discussed, these inputs also include the circulating levels of sex hormones generated by the gonads.

Once the peripheral input is received, a signal is generated from the hypothalamus, which is the same center we discussed in the four doors of the metabolism. This initial signal is a hormone called *gonadotropin releasing hormone*

(GNRH), which travels from the hypothalamus to the pituitary gland where it stimulates production of two important hormones called *gonadotropins*. These gonadotropins are called *luteinizing hormone* and *follicle stimulating hormone* (LH and FSH). LH and FSH then then stimulate the *gonads* in both males (testicles) and females (ovaries).

In males, when the LH signal reaches the testicles, it triggers production of the hormone *testosterone* while FSH is involved in sperm production and the hormone *inhibin*. In females, LH and FSH are responsible for *estrogen* and *progesterone* production, follicle maturation and ovulation. *Testosterone* and *inhibin* in males, and *estrogen* and *progesterone* in females send their signals back to the brain where they influence future GNRH production. It's essentially a feedback loop that informs itself and adjusts constantly. In a normal situation without any glitches, the *testosterone* and *inhibin* in males and the *estrogen* and *progesterone* in females send their signals back to the hypothalamus and pituitary gland. Based on their levels, the levels of GNRH from the hypothalamus and LH and FSH from the pituitary gland are adjusted up or down accordingly, based on whether more or less of the testicular or ovarian hormones are needed.

But this normally automatic process can become significantly disrupted in the case of metabolic dysfunction and glitches in the metabolic feedback loop.[4] Once this

4. Messini CI, K Dafopoulos, M Malandri, et al., Inhibitory Effect of Submaximal Doses of Ghrelin on Gonadotropin Secretion in Women. Hormone and Metabolic Research (2014), Vol. 46 No. 1: 36-40, doi: 10.1055/s-0033-1355388

occurs, fertility is interrupted due to either lack of reassuring input signals from the peripheral metabolic pathway, suppression of hypothalamic or pituitary responsiveness, insufficient pituitary stimulation of the gonads, or insensitivity of the gonads to pituitary hormone stimulation.

The hunger hormone ghrelin and the important hormone leptin (from the body fat) play a strong role in reproduction.[5] In males, *testosterone* produced in the testicles is released into the blood stream where it converts to free testosterone, the more activated form. On laboratory testing, the testosterone produced from the testicle is referred to as "total" testosterone, while the testosterone in the activated form is "free testosterone." In men with extra belly fat, total testosterone is often converted to excess estrogen. For some men this process perpetuates a cycle of excess estrogen and insufficient testosterone, leading to even more body fat distribution in female areas like belly, hips, and breasts. Ghrelin and estrogen can both similarly inhibit conversion of total testosterone to free testosterone, and on the flip side, leptin facilitates this conversion. In females, a similar process occurs where ghrelin can inhibit ovarian responsiveness to pituitary hormones and limit ovulation and estrogen production, while leptin can enhance the responsiveness, stimulating ovulation and estrogen production.

So common-sense factors dictate why our metabolism

---

5. Greenman Y, Rouach V, Limor R, et al. Testosterone is a strong correlate of ghrelin levels in men and postmenopausal women. Neuroendocrinology. (2009) Vol 89 No. 1:79-85. doi: 10.1159/000151768. Epub 2008 Aug 28.

The female fertility hormone pathway

©2015 Emily Cooper, M.D.

The female fertility hormone pathway disrupted

©2015 Emily Cooper, M.D.

The male fertility hormone pathway

©2015 Emily Cooper, M.D.

The male fertility hormone pathway disrupted

©2014 Diabesity Research Foundation
©2015 Emily Cooper, M.D.

determines our reproductive health to some extent. If there are signals of food scarcity or low body mass, whether accurate, as in anorexia, or wrongly perceived, as in metabolism glitches or Diet Fog (diet-induced biological adaptation that triggers starvation signals), a woman's ovulation and a man's testosterone production are sacrificed.

POLYCYSTIC OVARIAN SYNDROME (PCOS) IS NOT SO SIMPLE

There are many types of metabolic malfunctions linked to infertility in women but *polycystic ovarian syndrome* (PCOS), gets a lot of attention and is considered to be the most common cause of infertility in women.[6] Although there are definite objective markers linked to PCOS, like abnormal LH to FSH ratio, elevated testosterone and tiny cysts on pelvic ultrasound, I think of PCOS as a reversible condition with metabolic dysfunction as its root cause. The diagnosis can be a "wastebasket" diagnosis rather than a precise diagnosis in some cases because doctors do tend to group many women in this category even though there may be multiple factors contributing to their reproductive problems. PCOS can actually be due to a variety of causes, not just one, so it probably should be considered to be a collection of malfunctions with similar features and always rooted in metabolic dysfunction.

PCOS is usually associated with elevated testosterone and often another androgen, *dehydroepiandrosterone*

6. CDC April 16, 2015: What Causes Infertility in Women, http://www.cdc.gov/reproductivehealth/infertility/#d

sulfate (DHEAS). In PCOS ovulation is inhibited. Insulin resistance is often implicated, but what goes unnoticed is that other metabolic factors, such as high ghrelin or low leptin levels, can also trigger infertility.

There has been speculation about the cause of PCOS for decades. While some argue it's due to too much sensitivity to certain hormones, like insulin, others think it's due to lack of sensitivity to signals from the brain. A common explanation is that high testosterone interferes with female hormone production and action.

The traditional viewpoint is that PCOS is associated with insulin resistance. In my practice, insulin levels may be high or ghrelin may be elevated. And often there is a combination of these two excess hormones. It's possible that the powerful starvation signaler and neurotransmitter, *agouti-related protein* (AgRP) can be a culprit as well.

Many PCOS patients show high cortisol levels, often due to excess ghrelin, which influences cortisol production. And high ghrelin can compete and possibly interfere with leptin signals from the fat tissue to the brain, drowning out signals that the body is well nourished and replacing them with hunger signals. My clinical observation over many years is that the root culprit in PCOS is usually either hyperinsulinemia (high insulin levels) or ghrelin excess (and possibly elevated AgRP), or a combination of these imbalances. Since dieting raises ghrelin and AgRP levels, we may discover that PCOS can be caused or exacerbated by chronic dieting. Many post-anorexia patients do develop PCOS after their acute recovery period and it's not clear whether this condition preceded their eating disorder.

The important aspect that's often not relayed to patients is that PCOS is usually a reversible condition. With improvement in the underlying metabolic dysfunction, PCOS usually calms down and eventually resolves. But the reversal entirely hinges on correcting the underlying metabolic problem and contrary to popular thinking, this is usually not within a person's control with lifestyle strategies alone.

SIGNS AND SYMPTOMS OF PCOS VARY PERSON TO PERSON

- Acne
- Hirsutism (facial and abdominal coarse hair growth)
- Irregular periods
- Hair loss at temple areas
- Multiple tiny ovarian cysts (pelvic ultrasound)
- Infertility
- Abnormal weight gain
- Elevated DHEAS, testosterone, LH to FSH ratio, insulin, ghrelin

HYPOTHALAMIC ANOVULATION: REVERTING TO PRE-PUBERTY

One of the most common problems I see in women facing infertility is lack of ovulation due to a deficiency of LH, often in combination with very low leptin and high ghrelin levels. Remember that LH is an important hormone from the pituitary that signals the ovaries to ovulate. This condition is characterized by low LH and estrogen levels. In fact, this is the same type of scenario that we normally find in pre-pubertal girls, so in a sense this hormonal alteration is like reverting back to pre-puberty. And women with anorexia nervosa have such low LH and estrogen levels that they stop menstruating altogether. Many women with normal and even very high body weight actually stop menstruating for the same reason that underweight women do: a suppression of LH production from the pituitary gland leading to anovulation (lack of ovulation) or irregular ovulation.

Remember that the GNRH from the hypothalamus which tells the pituitary gland to release LH depends on reassuring signals from the peripheral metabolic pathway: insulin and GLP-1 that tell the brain there is adequate food supply, and leptin and amylin that say there is enough body weight. But ghrelin, the hormone that tells the brain the body is hungry, must not be elevated. As long as these factors are in balance, ovulation usually takes place without a problem. But if any combination of the above is off balance, ovulation can be in jeopardy.

If LH levels are suppressed in women with low body weight due to malnutrition, why would they also be deficient in so many women with high body weight? If you haven't guessed already, dieting is the primary reason for suppressed leptin, insulin, and amylin levels and elevated ghrelin levels. So chronic dieting, especially combined with underfueled exercise, is a primary cause of hypothalamic anovulation. Other reasons can be related to leptin resistance in which leptin levels are not low but the signal is not detected by the brain properly.[7]

LOW BLOOD SUGAR REACTIONS CAN BE A FERTILITY OBSTACLE

As in other areas affected by metabolic dysfunction, like obesity and pre-diabetes, it's also very common to see *hyperinsulinemic hypoglycemia* (HH) occur in men and women with infertility. In HH, insulin levels spike right after eating a meal, provoking a significant drop in glucose, most often 60 minutes after eating. Also true for many patients with obesity, this insulin spike and subsequent glucose crash can trigger elevations of hunger signals and suppression of leptin signals, which sets off alarms that can cause the body to store fat and also block

7. Hausman GJ, Barb CR, Lents CA. Leptin and reproductive function. Biochimie. (2012) Vol 94:2075-2081

reproduction. Patients dealing with HH not only feel tired or sleepy after meals but their symptoms can escalate to sweating, anxiety, nausea, headache, palpitations, and dizziness if the glucose levels plummet too far. For women with infertility who are experiencing this cycle, we can see a combination of metabolic consequences that become part of a vicious cycle of metabolic dysfunction, affecting their body weight and fertility with seemingly no end in sight.

Testing for HH requires what is called a *mixed meal tolerance test* MMTT, in which a mixed meal containing all food groups is consumed and lab tests for both glucose and insulin are run at 30-minute intervals following the meal for up to two hours.[8] The common advice for hypoglycemia is to eat small frequent meals throughout the day and avoid high glycemic carbohydrates. While eating frequently and including complex carbs, proteins and fats is a good idea, unfortunately, it's not always that easy to control hypoglycemia. Some people go to the extreme of cutting out carbohydrates altogether when dealing with low blood sugar, which is counterproductive, as it eventually depletes the glucose stores in the body, raises ghrelin, and suppresses leptin, leading to even more low-blood-sugar-episodes, excessive weight gain and persistent fertility problems.

---

8. Patarrão RS, Lautt WW, Macedo MP. Assessment of methods and indexes of insulin sensitivity. Rev Port Endocrinol Diabetes Metab. 2014;9(1):65–73

SO MANY WOMEN ARE JUST LOOKING FOR ANSWERS

I'd like to share the story of just a few of my female patients who struggled with infertility until their underlying metabolic dysfunction was addressed. They represent hundreds of women in my practice with similar stories. In the end, it was lab testing for metabolism markers that uncovered the culprits interfering with their ovulation and ability to conceive. And only then could an appropriate treatment plan be implemented that restored the fertility for these women.

TRACY

When I met Tracy, she told me that she had previously been diagnosed with PCOS and infertility and doctors had told her that if she wanted to become pregnant she needed to lose weight. But what we found was that the very things she had been doing to try to lose weight made fertility even further from her reach. In fact, in spite of the extra weight she was carrying, all the dieting left her body feeling too starved to ovulate.

Tracy had long-standing problems with weight gain and had tried numerous diet-and-exercise strategies but her weight never responded in a meaningful way. When her doctor recommended more rigorous diet and exercise, explaining that her infertility was tied to her higher body weight, she applied herself even more. But the more she dieted and the more she exercised, the more irregular her menstrual cycle became, and not only did she remain infertile, but she had not lost that extra weight.

Her blood tests revealed she was in Diet Fog with low leptin levels and high ghrelin levels. Because she had dieted and exercised so much in the past, her brain and body thought she was starving and started to fight back. As we've discussed, this is a common situation that eventually occurs for everyone on a diet. With chronic dieting, leptin, a hormone from the body fat which tells your brain your body has enough fat stores, decreases and the hunger hormone, ghrelin, from the stomach, which tells your brain your body is hungry, spikes. This imbalance convinced Tracy's brain that her body's weight and food supply were too low. It also interfered with her ability to ovulate, because when the brain thinks you're starving it won't allow the body to become pregnant. It's the body's way of protecting itself. As I've explained previously, we see this same condition in some extreme athletes and patients with anorexia. Only when Tracy stopped dieting and markedly reduced her exercise did her reproductive system gradually begin to normalize.

The metabolic details that explain how this happens involve certain hormones and chemicals we've talked about, like leptin, which stimulates ovulation, and ghrelin, which inhibits ovulation (and others we haven't mentioned, like kisspeptin and oxytocin). So many of these little talked about hormone messengers influence not only body weight but reproduction as well.

To have any chance of becoming pregnant, Tracy had to stop dieting and cut back on her workouts. She had already dieted for years and as a result she wasn't ovulating. It was hard for her to make the changes. She wasn't used to eating carbs at all, so when I asked her to eat bread she had a really difficult time.

After several months of consuming all food groups regularly six to eight times a day, including the carbohydrates which she had previously avoided, and taking medication to improve her metabolic hormone balance, her metabolism began to perk up and the hormones that regulate her ovulation started to normalize. As leptin levels increased and ghrelin levels decreased, her brain stopped worrying about starvation and allowed a key hormone, *luteinizing hormone* (LH), that triggers ovulation, to surge. This led to an increase in estrogen production, more normal periods, and eventually pregnancy! In fact, her estrogen level rose by ten times within six months.

Like so many patients, it was really hard for Tracy to do the opposite of what everyone had been telling her. She had spent years dieting and exercising. But all that

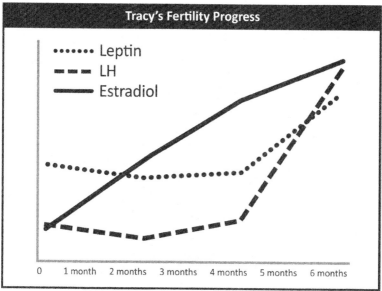

©2015 Emily Cooper, M.D.

did was make it harder to get pregnant and harder to lose weight! Because her body thought she was starving she couldn't get pregnant, but about a year later, it finally happened and now she has a beautiful baby boy!

Throughout her pregnancy lab tests show that Tracy's metabolism stayed on a good track. That she didn't have gestational diabetes was good news for both mom and baby in terms of future risk. She continued to eat regularly throughout her pregnancy and into the post-partum period. In the future, we'll need to make sure her metabolic hormones remain in balance because this problem can prevent potential future pregnancies and can also affect her health.

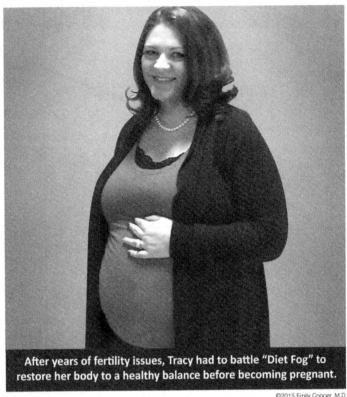

After years of fertility issues, Tracy had to battle "Diet Fog" to restore her body to a healthy balance before becoming pregnant.

I would love the change that led to Tracy's eventual pregnancy to happen more quickly for all my patients, but it really takes the body time to recover and get back on track. It usually doesn't happen overnight, and everyone's metabolism responds differently.

CHERYL

Take Cheryl, who had given up on pregnancy after seven years of trying everything, including extensive fertility treatments. She came to see me about her longstanding battle with weight, having never successfully lost weight for more than very short periods during the most extreme diets. Seven years earlier she had become pregnant as a result of fertility treatment, and during that pregnancy she gained over sixty pounds, though her baby weighed under six pounds at term. This information led me to believe that Cheryl's body thought she was starving during her last pregnancy and that was probably the reason that she was unable to conceive both then and now.

Cheryl's lab work showed that although her leptin levels were more than adequate her brain was not registering her leptin signal. This resistance to the leptin signal was one of the metabolic disruptions that she was experiencing, causing not only her body weight to climb—in spite of a healthy lifestyle—but also suppressing her LH levels, similar to what happens when leptin levels are too low. As a result, her ovulation was also suppressed. To her surprise, as soon as we started a treatment for her metabolism, she became pregnant within just a couple of months! So, unlike Tracy and most other patients, things turned around for Cheryl very rapidly!

HEIDI

It's not only patients with weight challenges who are dealing with metabolic dysfunction that disrupts their reproduction. Heidi, who was a competitive amateur rower and longtime endurance athlete, had come to see me for a VO-2max test, a type of fitness test which looks at the level and type of energy expended at rest and during exercise. She was planning to get married and hoped to become pregnant soon after. Because the testing showed that she was not combusting carbohydrates normally and because her resting metabolism showed an increased use of proteins for energy, rather than carbohydrates and fats, I suspected that if she stopped her birth control pills she might not have a normal menstrual cycle. Even though her weight was normal, these clues told us that her brain most likely thought her body was starving.

Sure enough, Heidi didn't see her menstrual cycle for a whole year after she stopped the birth control pills. Labs showed she had what is referred to in medicine as *hypothalamic amenorrhea*—similar to hypothalamic anovulation, but indicating that she did not menstruate on her own at all. But Heidi wasn't dieting! She ate three square meals and even some snacks but she simply underestimated her fuel needs to match her workouts. And a major culprit was that several workouts throughout the week took place early in the morning, on an empty stomach, before breakfast.

After working on tightening up her daily nutrition and cutting back the exercise, just as Tracy needed to do, Heidi's menstrual cycle finally returned. She fueled very reliably and did her best to keep things in balance. Unlike Tracy, Heidi didn't have any problems with obesity. This was largely due to genetic differences and she happened to have a very strong level of the key metabolic hormone MSH, which we discussed in previous chapters. MSH is the hormone that helps activate the receptor in the brain responsible for regulating the body's weight set point. So it's likely that along with her genetics, Heidi's strong MSH level kept her body weight in a normal range.

At first, she thought that playing tennis for hours wasn't really a workout because, after all, it was low key and her heart rate wasn't even that elevated. But she eventually realized that she needed to fuel all the physical efforts with great care in order for her body to turn her hormones back on. We used a synthetic form of a natural metabolism hormone to help her brain and ovaries see her body weight more clearly so it would really trust that she was now nutritionally secure. As a result, Heidi has not only had one healthy child but she just gave birth to a second!

REVERSING METABOLIC DYSFUNCTION REVERSES INFERTILITY

Tracy, Cheryl, and Heidi were each dealing with metabolic dysfunction that was impairing their fertility, and by addressing the underlying issues they, like dozens of other patients, have had successful pregnancies. We've talked about how metabolism glitches can occur in those who are genetically vulnerable. These glitches cause the brain to wrongly perceive starvation, triggering weight gain, and often affecting reproduction. And since chronic diets and underfueled exercise amplify the glitches, they add fuel to the fire and are a huge culprit. And this situation is so common!

If the body doesn't want you to become pregnant because it rightly (as in anorexia, underfueled exercise or deprivation dieting) or wrongly (due to genetic glitches) perceives starvation, then fertility treatment might not work. If it does work, then moms often gain a lot of weight in pregnancy due to lingering starvation signals and the body's attempts to further protect them from perceived starvation. This only amplifies with nursing, causing many moms to report weight gain in pregnancy that never comes off.

Researchers have also found that children born to moms who have undergone fertility treatments like *in vitro fertilization* (IVF)[9] are often found to have higher

---

9. Chen M, Norman RJ, Heilbronn LK. Does in vitro fertilisation increase type 2 diabetes and cardiovascular risk? Curr Diabetes Rev. (2011) Vol 7 No. 6:426-432

So what should I do if I am dealing with infertility?

- Sleep 8 hours
- Reduce cardio exercise
- Fuel all activity appropriately
- Eat all food groups every 3 hours
- Keep stress levels down
- Get a metabolic workup:

Women
insulin, leptin, ghrelin, glucose, LH, FSH, estradiol, testosterone by equilibrium dialysis, DHEAS, prolactin, cortisol, IGF-1, rule out post-meal hypoglycemia

Men
total and free testosterone, insulin, ghrelin, glucose, LH, FSH, estradiol, IGF-1, rule out post-meal hypoglycemia

©2015 Emily Cooper, M.D.

body weights as adults. I wonder if this is due to the effect of the IVF itself or to the fact that starvation signals which originally interfered with conception persisted in the mother throughout her pregnancy and were transmitted to her offspring.

Scientists have long studied how maternal undernutrition is thought to affect babies by causing amplification of gene changes in the fetal brain, possibly predisposing offspring to altered energy expenditure and glucose balance later in life.

Tracy, Cheryl, and many of my other patients who conceive after restoring their metabolic function haven't usually had excessive weight gain during pregnancy and their babies are born at normal birth weights. After their bodies had become appropriately reassured that they were not starving and it was safe to conceive, their metabolism usually stayed on a good track throughout the pregnancy.

Correcting metabolic dysfunction successfully reverses infertility in so many patients. And when a mom has lowered the levels of starvation signals in her own body, she shares her healthier environment with her developing baby.

CHAPTER 10

Science Holds the Answers

SO, IF DIET AND EXERCISE IS not an effective
long-term solution to overweight and obesity, then what
is? This is literally the $60 billion question—after all,
that's what the US diet industry is worth annually.

As we've previously discussed, science shows that
weight problems are associated with complex underlying
imbalances in the metabolic feedback loop. Accordingly,
treatments that repair, reset, and realign the feedback
loop are by far the most promising options that exist today. And the good news is that scientists who are working
on these types of solutions have made terrific progress in
the past two decades; we are already benefitting from their

discoveries and still we hope for more streamlined and innovative treatments to emerge over the next decade.

So, if science has the answers, why isn't anyone talking about them? In fact, researchers in this field are talking—it's just that most other people aren't privy to this information. Few people read journals with sexy names like *Disease Models and Mechanisms* or textbooks called "The Neurobiology of Obesity." In the meantime, millions get their fitness and health tips including weight-loss advice from popular magazines, commercials and other mainstream media sources.

I have wondered why the science of metabolism gets so little press. One reason may indeed be the growing diet industry, which permeates nearly every aspect of our daily life, drowning out the messages that science has to offer. People often experience sometimes dramatic short-term results on diets, and they believe that the next one will work as well or better—and they think the reason that they haven't been successful in keeping the weight off is because they didn't stick to the diet. They don't realize that cutting calories and food groups, and exercising as a means to long-term weight management, is flawed due to the inevitable biological adaptation that eventually causes the body to store more fat.

Another reason for the silence about metabolism's role in weight gain is that the pharmaceutical industry—

the industry that is working on treatments I'm talking about—is dragging its feet. This is understandable: the AMA and several other health organizations have now categorized obesity as a disease; in fact, "a multi-metabolic hormonal disease state," but many insurance companies still will not cover treatments related to obesity.Even if the pharmaceutical companies come up with safe, effective treatments that are easy to administer, there's a good chance that few healthcare providers will prescribe them and no insurance companies will pay for them. Fortunately, the federal government recently changed its policy so that obesity-related treatment must be covered for federal employees. I am hopeful that this will be the beginning of a trend and that commercial insurers will eventually adopt the same policy. The greatest impediment in moving from problem to solution is the widespread belief that obesity is a personal flaw rather than a medical condition. Only when the public and healthcare providers have embraced the scientific evidence that obesity is a medical condition can we really begin to routinely talk about treatment.

HISTORY REPEATS ITSELF

What I find truly fascinating about this area of medicine is that the most advanced and current scientific viewpoint of obesity is, in many ways, not new at all. In fact, as I explained in Chapter 5, it's actually close to one hundred years old. The leading endocrinologists and metabolic experts of the early 1900s recognized that diet and exercise were not a long-term "cure" for weight problems, and they believed the true solutions to addressing overweight and obesity would lie in hormonal treatments designed to realign the feedback loop. You may be surprised to hear that by the 1920s, these experts were writing that diet and exercise cures for obesity were already two decades outdated, and by the 1950s it was well established that diets slow metabolism and have significant limitations, even as a temporary solution. So what happened? Why has it taken so long for others to recognize this? The great minds of the 1920's were ahead of their time even though they didn't have ways to really measure what they observed. As the decades passed, scientists began to discover the reasons behind these early medical observations.

In the 1980s and '90s, several important metabolism-regulating hormones—amylin, leptin, adiponectin, and ghrelin—were discovered. This paved the way for even more discoveries about how the metabolism functions. And over the last decade, scientists who have studied the specific biochemical reasons why dieting causes metabolic slowdown have proven that diets leave a lasting fingerprint that promotes weight *regain.*

In Dr. Lisser's 1924 publication, *The Frequency of Endogenous Endocrine Obesity and Its Treatment By Glandular Therapy* he states:

> *I venture to predict that the supreme triumph will come in the end from the isolation of hormones specific for certain types of adiposity, just as the pinnacle of diabetic research was reached in insulin.*

Lisser's prediction of future solutions, based on the utilization of hormones and bioactive agents that are part of the metabolic feedback loop, illustrates his great insight into metabolism and weight issues. Even with just the limited science that was available at the time, he understood that effective treatment of obesity would only be possible when the specific hormones involved in the metabolic process were identified and isolated as part of a medical treatment. And it wasn't only Lisser who thought so: many prominent physicians of his time agreed. Dr. F.M. Pottenger, for example, had this to say in 1924:

> *A very large group of people suffer from obesity. It was formerly thought that this was due to overeating and lessened exercise. We now know, however, that there are certain glands of inter-*

nal secretion whose function influences greatly the shape and size of the body.

Lisser's and Pottenger's contemporary, Dr. N.W. Janney, also believed that endocrine issues triggered obesity in most cases:

One or two decades ago it seemed sufficient to recognize exogenous obesity, due to overeating and underexercise, and endogenous obesity, usually vaguely relegated to a "constitutional" or "familial" tendency . . . With accumulation of knowledge of the ductless glands, it has, however, become a certainty that an endocrine etiologic factor underlies the development of overweight in most cases, as Dr. Lisser's timely paper emphasizes.

Lisser and his colleagues rejected what they described as an already outdated view—that merely energy intake and expenditure governed weight regulation in obesity. Instead, they honed in on the concept of an underlying metabolic problem as a root cause of obesity. Their vision of a cure that focused on hormonal regulation of the fat tissue was incredibly insightful. But due to the complexity of this task, it has taken scientists nearly one hundred years to map the pathophysiology (abnormal physiology) of these underlying causes of obesity and translate that information into viable potential treatments.

When it comes to the subject of obesity, in spite of 100 years of scientific challenge to the status quo, most physicians today are not only unaware of perspectives expressed by esteemed clinicians from the 1920s, but they are not familiar with great discoveries in metabolism during our time. What is it about the subject of overweight and obesity that particularly seems to blind people to scientific truth? Much of the science is complex and counterintuitive, which may be a major reason the disconnect has perpetuated over an entire century!

OBESITY UNDER THE MICROSCOPE

During this ninety-year absence of effective medical treatment, the diet industry has blossomed into what it is today. Well-funded diet and exercise studies have been repeated over and over again at major universities, producing the same results: a lack of long-term effectiveness and slowing of the metabolic rate, which encourages weight regain. It's as though we believe if we conduct enough studies, the results will be different. What if we instead had funneled those resources into exploring novel concepts and potential treatments?

As my own practice has evolved, over the past decade in particular, I see that clinical evaluation and treatment of patients with obesity is a highly technical process. After taking a careful history, starting in the womb and including family history spanning generations, the next step is to essentially put the patient "under the microscope" to evaluate the metabolic system. While fifteen years ago measuring hormones like leptin, MSH and ghrelin just wasn't a possibility in a clinical setting, things have changed dramatically, improving diagnosis and treatment capability. Results of today's clinical lab tests reflect that weight problems are driven by metabolic problems.

Like any medical condition, patients who are particularly weight prone present with classic symptoms, display abnormal test results and respond to a targeted treatment. That constellation of findings in patients with obesity proves that obesity is a *multi-metabolic hormonal disease* state, as the AMA and AHA have stated. Diseases have classic symptoms, signs which are objective markers of dysfunction, and they respond to treatment that targets the dysfunction. Obesity is a disease and should be recognized as a disease.

My patients initially report symptoms of appetite irregularity, fatigue, unexplained weight gain or weight-loss resistance, and they show abnormal levels and functions of their metabolic feedback loop. Typical lab results indicate low leptin or adiponectin, abnormal glucose and insulin balance, low MSH, GLP-1 deficiencies, excessive neuropeptide Y and ghrelin, insulin resistance, and/or leptin resistance. In addition to these specific metabolism imbalances, I often see suppression of TSH, LH and ACTH, as we've discussed in the chapter on fertility. Male patients also show low total and free testosterone levels, while their estrogen levels are often elevated. A percentage of patients also present with metabolic syndrome, including abnormally high LDL particle counts, triglycerides with low HDL levels, elevated blood pressure, and pre-diabetes. The ability to objectively diagnose metabolic problems that cause obesity through lab testing is critical. If weight problems are diagnosed medically, the treatment focus shifts from merely targeting the weight with a short-term strategy, prescribing a diet or exercise plan, and instead moves toward treating the underlying metabolic malfunction.

While the availability of clinical tests has improved dramatically over the past decade, we still cannot readily test a patient's genes to identify genetic vulnerabilities: for example, the new FTO gene associated with obesity, or a genetic mutation of the MC4R, or other chromosomal information abnormalities. However, we *can* gain an impression of metabolic health from laboratory data and improve the function of the metabolic feedback loop through individualized medical treatments. Almost one hundred years after first being recognized by Lisser as the "supreme triumph" of obesity treatment, the dream of pinpointing the underlying hormonal causes of weight gain and using medications to address them has finally become a reality. Applying these strategies broadly so all physicians have the necessary knowledge and all patients have access will be the next great challenge.

THE COCKTAIL APPROACH

When I first began to evaluate my patients' metabolisms I recruited the best minds on my team to help create charts which listed identifiable factors in the scientific literature that affected every metabolic hormone and neurotransmitter. We searched for strategies to lower or raise leptin, lower ghrelin, raise GLP-1, and increase adiponectin, etc. I first looked at foods, supplements, and lifestyle strategies. I then examined medications, both detrimental and beneficial to metabolism. We tracked scientific publications for the most specific information about every aspect of metabolism. As you can imagine, this process resulted in the construction of huge charts and cross-references. Surprisingly, I found that even innocent everyday supplements like vitamin C could have a negative impact in a particular setting.

Initially, I tried putting my patients on supplements to raise adiponectin, lower ghrelin, or improve GLP-1. But over time I found that supplements had unpredictable responses, some beneficial and some unwanted. Compared to pharmacologic products, natural products, like supplements, lack specificity when used as a medicine. One benefit of synthesized medications is that they isolate a specific compound for a specific therapeutic benefit, and most have roots from substances found in nature. Over the years I found that due to the complexity of the metabolic system, in the vast majority of cases, pharmaceutical medication is safe and performs superiorly to supplements. In my own clinical approach, specific targeted supplements are a part of the treatment strategy but they are usually a supportive element rather than a primary player. Their role becomes a little more prominent when working with children as many medications are not studied in children and certain supplements have very good safety records, so although the efficacy is inferior, their safety profile does make them a good option if chosen carefully when treating youngsters.

The role of medications in obesity treatment is just beginning to be better understood. Metabolic problems are complex. Each patient needs a customized plan. Scientists have frequently reported that a "cocktail" approach, combining sophisticated medications to attack multiple glitches along the feedback loop, carries the most potential, since hormones act synergistically to improve metabolic function in a healthy metabolism. Even after applying a sophisticated medical treatment plan, in some cases the patient may also benefit from bariatric surgery, which, like medication, has a profound metabolic impact, at least initially. Fortunately, most of my patients have not needed to include surgery as part of their treatment approach, but in some cases where medical treatment effectiveness is limited, surgery can help break the gridlock. But since surgery does not permanently fix the underlying problem, medical treatment is an essential component if the goal is long-term metabolic health.

We are hearing more and more about the cocktail approach to obesity treatment. A recent article published in *Disease Models & Mechanisms* emphasizes that combination treatment is the most promising strategy for addressing weight problems:[1]

> *To succeed in developing drugs that control body weight to the extent seen following surgical intervention, it seems obvious that a new paradigm is needed. In future, this polytherapeutic strategy could possibly rival surgery in terms of efficacy, safety and sustainability of weight loss.*

1. R.J. Rodgers, M.H. Tschöp, J.P.H. Wilding, "Anti-obesity drugs: past, present and future," Disease Models & Mechanisms (September 2012), 5(5), doi: 10.1242/dmm.009621, PMCID: PMC3424459: 621–626.

The goal of any medical treatment should be to address what's causing the problem, not merely to mask the symptoms. If you had a headache and it kept coming back, wouldn't you rather try to find out why than simply take aspirin day after day as a temporary fix? Wouldn't you wonder what was causing the headache to recur? Weight problems are no different.

TREATING OBESITY AS A MEDICAL CONDITION

The new 2015 clinical guidelines for clinical treatment of obesity from the Endocrine Society have shifted dramatically in the direction of a more scientific approach.

The guidelines are groundbreaking, because for the first time using medication to treat obesity is now recommended above not using medicines. In other words, it's now considered good practice for doctors to prescribe medication to help patients who are trying to reverse their weight problems. Experts applaud these changes. Over the past two decades, researchers have shown that obesity is a complex condition and diets and exercise don't solve it for the majority of people.

But the new guidelines still do cling to old diet recommendations, disregarding the evidence that they can make matters worse. Although it's a welcome start, the guidelines don't discuss diagnosing the underlying problem, which makes it difficult to choose the best medicine for a patient. And one medication is recommended at a time, though research shows a cocktail approach may hold more promise, but it will take time to adopt this type of strategy. Finally, the guidelines recommend changing medication if weight loss is less than 20% per year but none of the medications have done that well in research studies!

So while the new guidelines are a promising step forward, improvements will be needed in the future. And it's going to take time for insurance companies to be on board, because most plans don't cover weight-related treatment. Perhaps legislation will change that. Federal employees are now covered for weight-related treatment and, at last, many organizations have claimed obesity is a disease. Now that clinical treatment guidelines have been established, doctors who follow these guidelines would be prescribing expensive medications that are not routinely covered by insurance. So if no generic alternatives are available, how will patients afford the recommended treatment?

PHARMACOLOGY PIPELINE

Contrary to common opinion, medical treatment does not work by suppressing appetite but is a way of bridging gaps and alleviating traffic jams in the metabolic feedback loop in order to restore the flow of normal and healthy signals. The result is a more even appetite and an increase in fat utilization and energy expenditure by the body. Once patients have made suffcient progress and their system returns to normalcy, in my experience medications usually can be gradually withdrawn. Several medica-tions have the potential to favorably impact the metabolic pathways. Next, we'll discuss some of those medications.

Metformin

Metformin, one of the oldest medications used to correct glitches in the metabolic pathway was discovered in the 1920s, and is still the most widely prescribed medication for type 2 diabetes today. It acts as a gatekeeper, regulating the pace at which the liver releases glucose between meals to prevent sudden surges of glucose into the bloodstream. In addition to its role in type 2 diabetes, it has also been widely used in pre-diabetes, insulin resistance and treatment of PCOS. It improves insulin sensitivity by controlling glucose levels and associated insulin response. It mostly works on the fasting metabolism because its main effect is to regulate the pace of hepatic (liver) glucose release into the blood stream during periods of fasting. A natural substance that acts like metformin is bitter melon, but to come close to the effectiveness of metformin you would have to consume a bushel a day and who knows what side effects that would present! Metformin is a very safe medication; however, since it's metabolized in the liver, testing liver function is important after initiating this medication.

Synthetic Hormones

Newer medications designed to address issues in the metabolic pathway include synthetic forms of the hormones involved. The correct terminology is *mimetics,* meaning these substances mimic the effects of natural hormones in the body. They are also called *receptor agonists,* meaning, like our own hormones, they can activate receptors in the metabolic pathway. They are very helpful as part of an overall treatment strategy for many patients because patients with obesity have been found to be deficient in several key areas of metabolism. Incretin mimetics are synthetic hormones that were first introduced to the market in 2005. This group of medications, now consisting of a half a dozen brands, mimic GLP-1, the hormone that is normally produced in the intestine. Like GLP-1, incretin mimetics help the brain see the nutrition in our food, regulate the pace at which food moves through our stomach and small intestine, and set the pace at which nutrients are absorbed into the bloodstream. They also regulate glucagon levels and the rate at which glucose is released from the liver during periods of fasting. They improve cardiometabolic indicators, such as blood pressure and cholesterol levels, as well as insulin sensitivity and visceral fat levels, and they have a favorable impact on ghrelin, NPY, and AgRP. In diabetics, incretin mimetics help the pancreas match the blood sugar with the appropriate amount of insulin by stimulating growth of new insulin-producing beta cells to replace some of those that no longer function. As you can see, this is a powerful and promising class of medications that has already made an enormous impact on diabetes and has begun to enter the mainstream of obesity medicine treatment as well.

A synthetic form of the hormone *amylin* was released in 2005. It improves insulin sensitivity and leptin sensitivity, allowing diabetic patients to use less insulin to control their blood sugar levels, and, similar to incretin mimetics, it regulates the pace of glucagon release. Amylin has a synergistic action with leptin: it augments the leptin signal in the brain, more clearly informing the brain of the body's weight status. In doing so, it reduces NPY and AgRP levels at Door One of the central metabolic pathway. The only amylin mimetic on the market is *pramlintide*. This medication has had little traction as an obesity treatment and its use has been normally confined to patients with diabetes treated with insulin. However, numerous studies have shown that when used in specific settings, it may offer an important treatment avenue for metabolic dysfunction. Interestingly, this medication has been tested in humans at eighty-five times the normal dose and has been found to have no toxicity. Since amylin helps the brain see the leptin signal, essentially it helps the brain see the body weight to improve the security signals along the metabolic feedback loop.

DPP-4 inhibitors, first released in 2006, can be used to inhibit the body's ability to break down GLP-1, thereby prolonging the effects of the GLP-1 the body produces on its own.

Other Metabolic Pathway Modifiers

The medication *topiramate* was discovered in 1979 and has been on the U.S. market since 1996. Originally developed to help prevent migraine headaches, topiramate's effect upon weight regulation has now been studied for many years. Although the exact mechanisms of its action are unknown, it is thought that its effectiveness is primarily due to its favorable impact on NPY activity at Door One in the central metabolic pathway.

Bupropion increases activity at Door Two of the central metabolic pathway and production of the hormone POMC which converts to ACTH. If you remember the central pathway Door Two mechanism, ACTH is the precursor to MSH. Bupropion does not directly increase MSH but it improves the levels of MSH precursor hormones to help improve the potential for MSH production. It is a component of two new obesity medications, one new on the market and one still in development: *Contrave,* which consists of bupropion and a medication called naltrexone, which augments bupropion's metabolic action by assisting in the conversion of ACTH to MSH; and still in development is *Empatic,* which combines bupropion with zonisamide, a medication that is similar to topiramate but whose mechanism is thought to be different and possibly more impactful by not only targeting NPY but also affecting AgRP favorably with less side effects than topiramate. *Lorcaserin,* a medication released in 2013, also activates Door Two ACTH production, but via a different mechanism than bupropion. This is one medication in obesity treatment that is newly developed, not one that stems from older medications that we have been familiar with for years. It has passed the FDA safety trials, however, more time is needed to see how it performs clinically and what its potential risks are.

Phentermine, an appetite suppressant, and *orlistat,* a fat-absorption blocker, are also used in weight regulation. While phentermine may have action that impacts Door Two function, it's not clear whether it primarily works by suppressing appetite, rather than improving metabolic function in the long term. An FDA approved medication, *Qsymia*, combines *phentermine* with *topiramate*. *Orlistat* blocks fat absorption from the GI tract, so it can be considered the least sophisticated medication in the group. It is unlikely to have long-term benefit and inhibits absorption of fat soluble vitamins and causes oily loose stools.

PHARMACOLOGIC INVENTIONS ON THE HORIZON

The next decade will be very exciting for healthcare providers and patients as new treatment options become available. Researchers are developing synthetic versions of additional receptor agonists (hormone mimetics) and pharmacologic tools to help regulate the metabolic feedback loop. MSH, adiponectin, oxyntomodulin, and PYY are all being studied, as well as blockers and supporters of specific functions along the feedback loop. Unfortunately, a couple of tracks that were under development appear to have become dead ends for logistical reasons, including the combination of synthetic leptin with amylin (pramlintide) and an immunization that reduces elevated ghrelin. Scientists are still working on an immunization against adenovirus 36, which is a virus implicated in triggering obesity in susceptible individuals. And they continue to study new ways to simulate "brown fat," which is highly metabolically active. Development of Door Four receptor (MC4R) agonists, i.e., MSH mimetics, are highly anticipated as we move into the next decade.

In combination with the medications that are already on the market, these promising new potential treatments may address most of the common glitches in the metabolic pathway. Genetic testing is also on the horizon and will eventually be useful in understanding individual root causes and developing more targeted treatments. As science continues to progress—and it's happening at an amazingly fast pace—our ability to clinically measure the body's metabolic hormones and apply more effective treatment will only improve.

BARIATRIC SURGERY

Many physicians today are promoting bariatric surgeries, such as gastric bypass, vertical sleeve, and lap band, as a way to not only lose weight but also reverse diabetes. These surgeries do have *some* benefits: they produce some of the most impressive initial weight-loss rates of any treatment available. Although the majority of patients experience weight regain post-op, they usually don't regain *all* of the weight lost.

Bariatric procedures have been largely categorized as restrictive—meaning the size of the stomach is reduced, or malabsorptive—meaning that nutrient absorption from the gut is reduced. The lap band and vertical sleeve are restrictive while the gastric bypass is both restrictive and malabsorptive. The current data shows that the lap band has not been effective for most patients over the long term, while the Vertical Sleeve Gastrectomy (VSG) is gaining in popularity because of its low complication risk and high success rate. The VSG used to be performed as part of a more radical procedure and has now become a routine procedure on its own. The Roux-en-Y Gastric Bypass (RYGB) has been a standard procedure for decades now and while the success rate is high, since absorption of nutrients is affected, there are more potential long-term risks and complications. Both the VSG and RYGB procedure are performed laparoscopically .

Bariatric surgeries like the RYGB and VSG are shown to favorably alter many of the hormones disrupted by both original metabolic problems and prior diets.

Many of my patients who have undergone bariatric procedures have come to see me for help with weight regain or blood sugar regulation issues in the months or years following their surgery. In the short term, many of them lost a great deal of weight—100, 150, or even 200 pounds within a couple of years, especially those who had a VSG or Roux-en-Y gastric bypass procedure. And the surgery does, in fact, bump many patients out of diabetes and back into pre-diabetes, insulin resistance, or even normal status in some cases. In the majority of these cases, however, at least a portion of the lost weight is eventually regained.

And surgery often doesn't permanently reverse the underlying cause of the weight problem. Since surgeons advise patients to remain on a lifelong diet following surgery, this can eventually impact the metabolism like any diet, triggering the body's weight-defense system and leading to weight regain. Many patients eventually develop Diet Fog and their Metabolic Storm returns, causing them to regain a significant amount of weight and, in some cases, triggering a return to diabetes. In fact, due to these issues, 85% of post bariatric surgery patients are still in the obese weight range ten years after surgery. Therefore, regardless of the procedure type, the initial weight loss following bariatric surgery is most often followed by regain. Most patients will have lost 15% of their body weight ten years later, but up to 25% regain nearly all or more of the weight they initially lost. Medical treatment offers great potential for most patients but there are some patients that could benefit from combining surgical and medical treatment because they don't responde to either one of these approaches alone. An appropriate evaluation of the metabolic system is critical to identifying those who are potentially good surgical candidates, and medical follow up after surgery is essential to as-

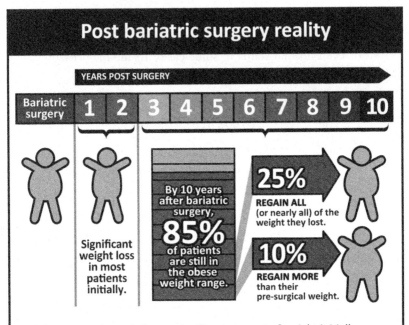

Post bariatric surgery reality

While most patients do lose a significant amount of weight initially after bariatric surgery, there is usually some weight regain that begins after a few years.

By 10 years after bariatric surgery, 85% of patients are still in the obese weight range. For patients in Karen's weight range pre-operatively, 25% regain nearly all the weight they lost and nearly 10% end up at an even higher weight than their pre-surgical weight.

suring a better long-term outcome. Ultimately, solving life-long metabolic issues requires an individualized approach, and it can't happen overnight

Additional Procedures and Devices

A new procedure that show promise is the VBLOC device, which regulates the communication pathway from the gut to the brain and back. This nerve pathway is called the *vagus nerve bundle* and is located at the upper part of the stomach. Remember that dozens of signals travel from the gut to the brain to inform the brain about the status of the body's nutritional condition, so this device attempts to optimize these signals. This procedure is done under general anesthesia laparoscopically and carries low risk. The device is meant to be a temporary device and short-term studies showed lingering weight loss maintenance after the device was removed. However, patients were only tracked for several months so this is not an indicator of long-term success rates. The weight loss rate observed over one year is more modest than other surgical procedures, but due to its safety and effectiveness, the device gained FDA approval in the US in 2015. Other devices are being investigated, include those that can potentially be inserted endoscopically rather than surgically, and that create a pressure sensation in the upper stomach in an attempt to influence the nerve pathway from the gut to the brain. These non-surgical devices are in early development and are not likely to be viable FDA approved devices for at least five years.

CHAPTER 11

WHAT DOES MEDICAL TREATMENT LOOK LIKE IN REAL LIFE?

THE FOLLOWING EXAMPLES show what happens when medical treatment based on science is combined with a non-diet approach to resolve metabolic problems that cause excess body weight.

REVERSING DIABESITY: JANET'S STORY

When Janet first came to visit me at age 50, she had significant obesity. She used to run marathons but had gradually gained weight over a number of years after she was

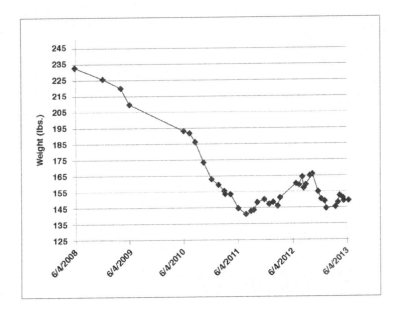

placed on medications for depression. She was unaware that she already had type 2 diabetes which we discovered at her first visit. She was so afraid to gain weight that she barely ate anything—but she still kept gaining. When we met, she was on so many medications that had so many side effects that she could hardly keep her eyes open. By the time she reached me she could barely get up off of the couch. When I asked her about her goal in working with me, I was shocked when she told me, "I want to be a competitive swimmer."

Once we began medical treatment Janet's hormonal settings gradually began to change. Within several months of adjusting medications, eating more regularly, and be-

Janet originally had type 2 diabetes and metabolic syndrome. After several years of treatment not only did she reverse diabetes and lose the excess weight, she also reached her dream of becoming a competitive swimmer

©2015 Emily Cooper, M.D.

ginning to address her metabolic problems, Janet's health had markedly improved. She was feeling much better. Although her body was initially resistant to weight loss, we worked on building her fitness, fueling each workout well so that her body's weight defenses would not activate. Within three years, in line with her goals, Janet actually entered her first swim competition. Over the next couple of years, changes in medication and additional correction of her underlying metabolic problems eventually led to steady weight loss.

Today, Janet has reached a normal weight and body-fat percentage, and she no longer has diabetes or even pre-diabetes. She has been free of diabetes for five years and has maintained a normal body weight for the past three years—and she's done so while eating more regularly than before we began treatment. She has met her goal of swimming competitively, and she now dreams of one day swimming the English Channel. Recovery didn't happen overnight for Janet, but after years of consistent treatment, she has experienced remarkable improvements in her health.

LILLY

Lilly had weight problems most of her life. She had a history of extreme dieting, and her weight issues increased

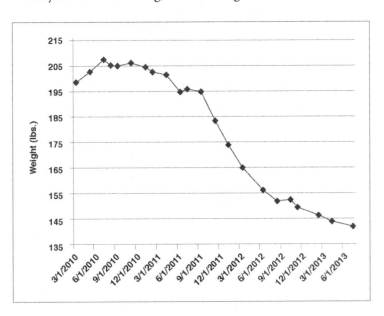

when she began to attend grad school. It took about a year to reverse her Diet Fog and then control her leptin resistance, but in the past two years her blood tests have shown improvement and her body weight has gradually and persistently dropped. Solely through realigning her metabolic feedback loop, Lilly's weight has been brought down to a normal range.

LAUREN

Lauren, a college student and professional cyclist, had a history of struggling with her weight. In spite of her heavy exercise load, she dieted constantly in an attempt to keep her weight from climbing. Before I met her, she had suffered an injury and had been treated with steroids,

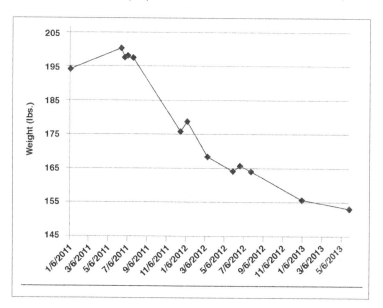

which contributed to rapid weight gain. Lauren's blood test showed significant Diet Fog. She had an initial weight increase while we dismantled her extreme dieting behavior, which was very frustrating for her, but once the Diet Fog cleared and we could address the underlying cause of her weight problem—insulin resistance—Lauren experienced steady weight loss. She is now maintaining a normal weight range, fueling her body well, and successfully competing again.

MADDY

Before seeing me, Maddy, age 17, had battled weight problems since early childhood. Her mother was very concerned because she was doing everything "right" but

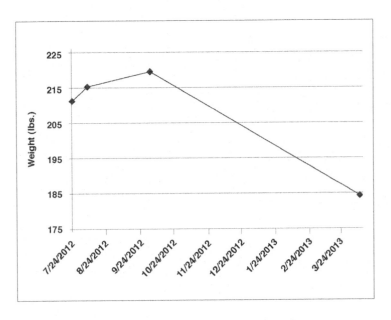

getting nowhere. Finally, Maddy's mother brought her to see me. Maddy's lab tests showed extreme Diet Fog. After she stopped exercising and started eating foods that she loved for the first time in her life, we identified the underlying problem: insulin resistance. With medical treatment, Maddy's weight has declined at a steady pace, and based on her lab work and progress so far, I am confident it will continue to do so with regular medical follow up.

RACHAEL

Before coming to see me, Rachael strictly followed a 1,200- to 1,400-calorie diet. A typical meal was chicken breast, salad, and steamed vegetables. Once a day she might allow herself a scoop of brown rice—but no dessert. She also

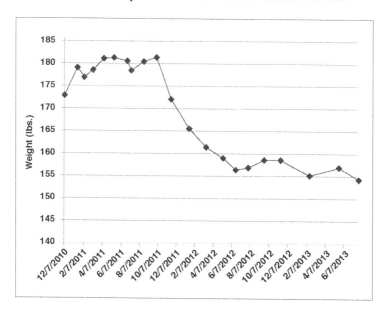

exercised heavily—often two to three hours a day, participating in a boot camp program or training for a triathlon.
Still, she was overweight, and her weight was steadily increasing in spite of her efforts.

Today, Rachael eats nutritious food, but she doesn't
count calories or restrict her eating. In fact, she eats
mashed potatoes, bread, maple bars, and chocolate cake
when she wants to—foods that were strictly off limit to
her for years. Rachel did not exercise during most of
her treatment, especially at first, so that her metabolism
could recover from Diet Fog. Following this protocol, not
only did her cholesterol and blood pressure fall into optimal ranges, but she lost a significant amount of weight.

ULTRAMAN: A REAL LIFE STUDY IN EXTREMES

Brian is a competitive triathlete, but was gaining weight
in spite of very careful eating and heavy training. He had
a big goal—to be one of a small group of people who
have successfully finished an event called the Ultraman.
The Ultraman is such a rigorous triathlon that it makes
Ironman look easy! It actually finishes off with a double
marathon! His training consisted of brick workouts with
bike and run sessions back-to-back and waking up at the
crack of dawn to meet his swim coach.

Brian's career is all about numbers and he's meticulous about keeping track of his training numbers: weight, food intake, heart rate and speed. So, when he saw that the standard calories-in/calories-out formula wasn't tracking—he was gaining weight, when according to normal calculations he should have been losing—he knew something was drastically wrong. In spite of training 20 hours a week and very careful eating, his weight continued to climb. Watching his weight escalate after his first major training race and Ironman event, he decided to seek answers and came to see me.

We started with testing his fitness to see what was happening metabolically during exercise. Exercise testing uses a system of measuring gas exchange within the content of the exhaled air, which tells not only how much fuel is burned but what type of fuel is burned: carbohydrates, protein, or fat. First we tested Brian's metabolism at rest. This showed that instead of burning about equal amounts of carbohydrates and fats, Brian was burning too much protein for energy.

Proteins are critical for the body to preserve because muscles, tendons, bones and important immune-system components are made of protein. In fact, the body normally conserves protein and burns carbohydrates and varying amounts of fat from excess adipose stores to get energy to keep the body operational. Only when fuel isn't available are proteins burned, and essentially borrowed from the immune system and from lean mass until these debts can be paid back after the next meal. If not replenished, this can lead to loss of lean mass and slowing of the metabolism. This finding was a clue that Brian's body was likely facing food scarcity in spite of his weight-gain trend.

We then tested Brian's metabolism during exercise, his ability to sprint, his high-level endurance and his low-level endurance as he moved from easy exertion to his most rigorous effort. Based on the testing, Brian had very little sprint capacity or high-level endurance capacity, mainly because he wasn't combusting carbohydrates powerfully enough as the physical work intensified. He felt like he couldn't go a step further even though he had not actually reached his own physiologic max.

Carbohydrates are the key nutrients that power high-intensity exertion and give athletes their speed. If something isn't working with carbohydrate combustion in the muscles, a person's higher effort levels spanning the top 10 or even 20 heartbeats of the entire heart-rate range could become inaccessible. In fact that's what happened to Brian.

Lab work helped shed light on the cause of these issues. Brian's anorexigenic hormones, like leptin and insulin, were suppressed, and his orexigens, ghrelin and NPY were elevated. Contrary to what people would expect, as his training increased he developed pre-diabetes. While he was eating what he thought was enough to fuel his training, it really wasn't sufficient to match his energy output. The more he trained, the more his ghrelin increased. Ghrelin is the hormone produced in the stomach that tells the brain that the body is hungry. So every time he worked out, the ghrelin levels would increase—eventually to a level so high that it caused his brain to panic and tell the body to store fat for protection against starvation. Scientists refer to this as *biological adaptation* and why diet and exercise are not a proven solution for obesity.

With the increasing training that Brian was facing, I was concerned. Sometimes hard training can backfire metabolically by triggering or amplifying a fear of starvation throughout the body. This may lead to glucose imbalances and decreased testosterone in men, reduced metabolic rates, elevated blood pressure and increased body fat stores—all issues that were already developing for Brian. But completing his goal of Ultraman was important to him because it was a tribute to someone he lost who had been very close to him.

Like Brian, I see lots of athletes ranging from recreational to World Champions who are experiencing symptoms related to metabolic dysfunction. The primary risk for athletes is that they can very easily end up with a mismatch of energy intake to expenditure. When this happens, it eventually leads to multiple metabolic problems including abnormal body fat gain and muscle loss and alteration of reproductive hormones. This condition is often referred to as *overtraining syndrome* which is simply an excess of starvation signals and a deficit of leptin and other nutritional security signals. This causes disruption of the central metabolic pathway and, as in obesity, a drastic drop in testosterone for men, and a drop in estrogen for women.

We monitored Brian's system as he boosted his nutritional intake so that his intake matched expenditure more closely. We used medication that mimics a key hormone that helped reassure his brain that he was carrying enough body weight. We also had to block some of the endorphins his body produced, since endorphins can obstruct metabolic function. He diligently consumed hundreds of calories per hour while he exercised and got plenty of sleep. He ate lots of carbs. By the time he reached the start line of the Ultraman, his body fat percentage was in the optimal range, his weight was in balance and he was off the medication. He could reach his maximal heart rates and he had improved his fitness.

SWIM 6 MILES, THEN BIKE 260 MILES, THEN RUN 52 MILES AND GAIN BODY FAT?

To his astonishment, something unexpected happened during the Ultraman competition. His body actually *gained* fat mass during the grueling three day race. During the race, he wasn't able to keep up with the robust caloric intake that he stuck to during training, so his body quickly began to store more fat for protection against perceived starvation, all due to *biological adaptation*.

You would never think that training for some of the most difficult races in the world could lead to gaining weight and developing pre-diabetes? And who would think that it was possible to actually *gain* body fat while expending all that energy and working so physically hard. But Brian's body reacted like Kate's did when she went from dieting and basic fitness training to Ironman, and also like Margaret, a medal-winning Olympian who trained at the highest level of elite performance but always fought extra weight. Their stories all illustrate that the metabolism is one of the most powerful biological systems in nature. It's a complicated system of checks and balances and when a glitch occurs it throws everything out of whack.

Why did it happen to Brian? Brian had weight problems when he was young, so his system had some built-

Brian's Ultraman Race Weekend

August 3 - 6:27 am

Duration:
3:45:30
Distance:
6.2 mi

August 3 - 10:18 am

Duration:
6:06:12
Distance:
90 mi

August 4 - 6:56 am

Duration:
10:05:55
Distance:
171.4 mi

August 5 - 6:58 am

Duration:
11:48:10
Distance:
52.4 mi

Total: 320 miles

in vulnerability that scientists call being "weight prone," which is thought to be up to 70% genetic. Combining the low fuel intake and the high fuel expenditure from all the training created a huge trigger for this particular metabolic dysfunction. But it doesn't take extreme training like Brian's to trigger the brain to tell the body to hold on to fat. Studies show that even after just a single endurance workout, some men's ghrelin levels increase 12% and for women that number jumps to as high as 24%!

The best defense, especially for those with genetics that put them at risk for obesity, is to get plenty of sleep, even an extra hour, and to keep up with all food groups throughout the day. During workouts, making sure to take in enough calories and carbohydrates is essential to preserving normal metabolic function.

If diet and exercise didn't work for Kate, who was training nearly twenty hours per week and competing in Ironman events, and Brian, who was training for and competing in the Ultraman, what hope is there for everyone else? What better way to illustrate what science has been telling us for decades than with their stories?

LISA

Lisa, 42, started dieting at age 12. She had some short-term success losing weight but began to gain rapidly after quitting smoking and going through a stressful move. Lisa joined a gym, worked out regularly, watched what she ate, and avoided carbohydrates. "I have tried everything! I'm in better shape than ever but now I'm heavier than I've ever been," Lisa said with exasperation. Smoking lowers the metabolism blocker, neuropeptide Y (NPY), so while she was smoking, her metabolism problems were masked. When Lisa stopped smoking her metabolic problems became difficult to manage. Fortunately, she responded to a minimal amount of medication which reversed her un-

Lisa Before

- Over 200 lbs.
- All time high body weight
- Carbohydrate depletion
- Exercising regularly
- Diet Fog (low leptin)
- Insulin resistance

Lisa After

- Medicine for insulin resistance
- Eat all food groups, including carbs at every meal
- Stop exercise temporarily
- Work on sleep
- Don't diet!

©2015 Emily Cooper, M.D.

derlying metabolic dysfunction and she has maintained a normal weight for several years.

DAVID

David, 58, came to see me to find out why he couldn't lose weight and why he felt "off." I found he had full-blown type 2 diabetes and metabolic syndrome. David had no idea he had these conditions or that his weight was a symptom of a much bigger underlying problem. He had high blood pressure, high cholesterol with plaque in his arteries, and his HBA1C was 8.8 (normal is 4.8-5.6). Now

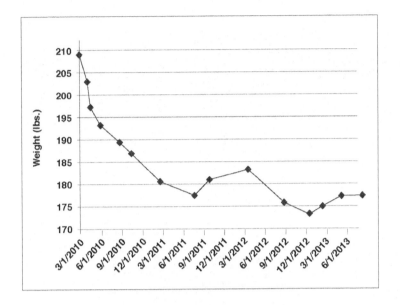

David is full of energy. His HBA1C is 5.9 and his blood pressure and cholesterol are in the lowest risk ranges.

BILL

Bill, six feet tall and 52 years old, came into my office with a stubborn weight problem and intense sugar cravings. I found that his weight problem was a symptom of a deeper medical issue. He had undiagnosed metabolic syndrome with insulin resistance and pre-diabetes, high cholesterol and LDL particles, and increased abdominal fat. Bill now has normal blood sugar levels, normal cholesterol and LDL levels, and normal blood pressure. Although his weight loss is moderate in terms of pounds, Bill's body composi-

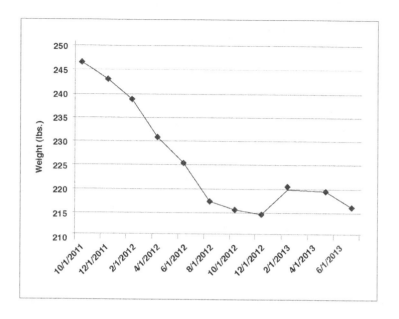

tion has improved significantly. We used a cocktail of medications to reverse Bill's stubborn metabolic dysfunction. He is doing so well that we are going to taper off some of the medications soon.

DANA

Dana, who is now 19 years old, first came to me as an adolescent after attending a diet boot camp to lose weight. She lost weight rapidly at the camp but eventually the weight began to creep back even though she was counting every calorie and exercising regularly. I found that Dana was in extreme Diet Fog. She was chronically tired, her menstrual cycles had stopped, she suffered several stress fractures and

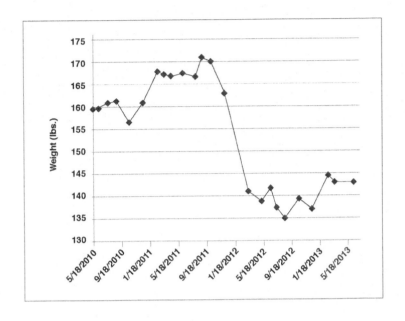

had low bone density. Dana's lab work showed that she had what essentially looked like anorexia caused by her diet-and-exercise program. It took about a year for her to come out of Diet Fog. The best we could do was to minimize the gain and stabilize her weight until, by eating regularly and abstaining from exercise, she came out of the Diet Fog. At that point, Dana's labs showed that insulin resistance was the root cause of her weight problem. After treating and reversing the insulin resistance, Dana's metabolism works normally. She has tapered off of insulin resistance treatment and remains on only a small amount of medical support—which soon will not be needed. The most important fact is that when she first came to my office Dana was literally starving and counting every calorie while gaining weight. Now she is eating freely, is far more nourished, and has a stable weight and metabolism.

BETTY

Betty, 65, suffered from knee arthritis and was unable to walk without a cane. She wanted more than anything to be able to play with her grandkids and have enough stamina to get through the day. Betty reported a long-standing history of obesity. She said, "When I was just 14, I had to starve myself to get my weight to go down at all." She had irregular hunger and satiety symptoms, often finding herself waking up in the middle of the night hungry. I found Betty had metabolic syndrome with high cholesterol, high blood pressure and pre-diabetes. Betty's excess weight was

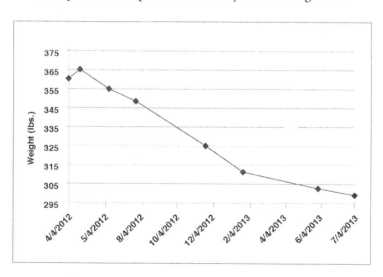

a symptom of underlying metabolic dysfunction. By focusing on regular eating, not dieting, and medically treating the underlying metabolic problems, Betty's health issues have finally begun to significantly resolve, her symptoms have disappeared and her weight is steadily declining. She is enjoying time with her grandchildren and has much more stamina.

KAYLA

Kayla struggled with weight problems for as long as she could remember. She spent years with crashing energy levels and an irregular appetite, and went on diet after diet trying to lose weight. As an adult she exercised and ate nutritiously, yet in spite of her efforts she found herself at an all-time high body weight and decided to undergo gastric bypass surgery. She lost a great deal of weight initially, exercising regularly and staying on a strict diet. But after five years she began gaining in spite of her efforts. So she ate less and less and exercised more and more but was devastated when she continued to gain weight. She experienced severe energy crashes that caused her to literally pass out on a regular basis. She had to pull over while driving because she felt so sleepy. She felt desperate and fearful.

Kayla's lab work showed that she was experiencing extreme drops in blood sugar every time she put something in her mouth, whether a balanced meal or a small nutritious snack. She felt dizzy and sweaty and her heart would race. Kayla didn't realize that these were symptoms of very low blood sugar (glucose) reactions. In fact we discovered that she had *hyperinsulinemic hypoglycemia* (HH). Her insulin levels were spiking and blood sugar levels were dropping to more than 20 points below the bottom of the normal *fasting* range and these drops were occurring *after* she ate! We tested her blood sugar levels throughout the day and night and found that they were also dropping to severely low levels while she was asleep. She began to realize that the symptoms were similar to what she had experienced as a child in the beginning of her battle with obesity.

She was shocked to learn that this very problem was the key reason that she was overweight in the first place and the bariatric surgery hadn't permanently fixed the underlying problem. Many physicians believe that the bariatric surgery itself is the cause of the blood-sugar problem, but studies show that reversing the gastric by-pass procedure does not correct the hypoglycemia. Also, if the bariatric surgery caused the problem, why would Kayla be having low blood-sugar reactions when she was sleeping, not only when eating a meal? And, what is most important, why would she have had similar symptoms as a child? And Kayla represents dozens of other patients I have seen with the same findings after surgery, and recall-ing the same symptoms earlier in their life. And they re-present hundreds of patients I see who have not under-gone surgery who also present with HH and obesity.

The reason that hypoglycemia causes weight gain in weight-prone people is that the extreme drops in blood sugar cause very strong starvation signals to the brain, altering hormone levels and neurotransmitters, causing the body to store fat for protection. These alterations include suppression of leptin and elevation of ghrelin, NPY, and AgRP. Most bariatric surgeons are taught that gastric bypass surgery reduces ghrelin levels permanent-ly; however, some of the highest ghrelin levels I have seen in my practice have been found in patients who have had gastric bypass surgery years prior. Unfortunately, re-searchers only studied these hormone changes for the first six to twelve months post surgery and, as we know, though surgery produces radical improvements in hor-mones initially, these changes revert towards baseline levels over time.

From the first day I met Kayla, I told her she had to stop dieting forever or we would never be able to cor-rect her problem. Like many patients, it was hard for her to trust initially, but now medical treatment has cor-rected most of Kayla's metabolic dysfunction and the ex-cess weight, which was a symptom, has reversed. She has

Kayla

©2015 Emily Cooper, M.D.

reached a normal weight for the first time in decades and has maintained that easily for a few years.

We are hopeful that by preventing dieting and supporting her now stronger metabolism she will have healthy blood sugar reactions and maintain a normal weight for the rest of her life.

RANDI

When Randi first came to see me she was really skeptical of my approach, but a friend insisted she investigate to see if there was a medical cause of her weight problem. She told me that she was only five pounds at birth, though full term, and her own experience since she entered puberty was that her body had always held on to extra weight. She said that she weighed 130 pounds at age 12 and by age 13 she had grown an inch and gained 80 pounds to 210. Over the years she tried every diet and had even lost and gained 100 pounds three times! She had given up on dieting at this point and her weight was stable around 290 lbs.

Her initial labwork showed metabolic syndrome with insulin resistance, a high number of small, sticky LDL cholesterol particles, high triglycerides and elevated blood pressure. Like Kayla, she had *hyperinsulinemic hypoglycemia* (HH) after eating (post meal insulin spikes and blood sugar crashes). But unlike Kayla, Randi never had bariatric surgery. Since the MC4 receptors (Door Four) strongly influence insulin levels, I've always assumed that hyperinsulinemic hypoglycemia could be linked to dysfunction of the MC4 receptors. The low blood sugar crashes were preventing her leptin from normalizing. In fact, her leptin was suppressed. In other words, her fat tissue was secreting much less leptin than normal, thus hiding most of her body's fat stores from her brain.

Very rapidly, with treatment of her metabolic dysfunction, Randi's LDL particles dropped over 1000 points and her triglycerides improved. We worked to stablize her post-meal glucose levels and prevent them from dropping.

Randi

©2015 Emily Cooper, M.D.

Once that improved, her leptin levels began to perk up. She lost weight rapidly in spite of very high neuropeptide Y (NPY) levels. This led me to believe that her MC4 receptors that regulate weight balance were functioning well during the time the weight was dropping. Fortunately, her ghrelin levels were not too elevated. Randi continued to make progress on the health and weight front. In fact, within 20 months she had lost 120 lbs!

But to my great surprise, we discovered that she has a rare genetic condition that causes her Door Four (MC4 receptors) to be deficient, with only half of the receptors actually working! So my previous assumption that she had stellar MC4 receptors was not really true. At this point I realized how amazing it really was that she had made the progress that she did in the short time that she did. MC4 receptor deficiency is the underlying problem in about 2-4% of all people with obesity. I was astonished to hear this news because Randi had been so responsive to treatment though most of the research papers published about this condition state that there is no current treatment available. We are hopeful that the weight will not return as long as Randi keeps her NPY, ghrelin and AgRP levels down to a minimum so that her working MC4 receptors can be activated without interference. This means that in addition to medications to support her metabolic feedback loop, she needs to continue to refrain from dieting and try to eat as regularly as she can and get enough sleep every night. Randi's challenging (but so far successful) case gives hope for every patient with metabolic dysfunction.

But not everyone's body responds smoothly

I wish everyone was a fast responder like Randi, but it's just not so in real life. Sometimes, in spite of all the efforts on the part of the patient, and the best treatment that medicine has to offer, we still cannot succeed in repairing the metabolic feedback loop, or the response can be painfully slow.

At a medical lecture I gave where Randi's case was one of two that I presented, a physician in the audience asked to what did I atrribute her great success? Was it that I somehow was brilliant with her care compared to other patients that might not respond as rapidly?" I answered that the main difference was not that I was a genius and constructed her treatment perfectly or differently than I would the others, but that the difference in response between one patient and another is really a matter of individual patient factors. No two patients are alike.

Response to treatment is influenced by past dieting history, time since last extreme dieting, exercise history, medications, lifestyle factors like environment, work and sleep schedules, and genetic and childhood factors. From my experience, the less dieting and exercise history the more responsive patients tend to be and the more extreme dieting and exercise history, especially if recent, then the more difficult it can be to achieve a healthy metabolism in a shorter time frame. Since Randi had not dieted for years before seeing me, maybe that played a part in her success. Indeed her brother, who is an avid athlete and meticulous with his diet, lost only 25 pounds in the time she lost 120. Almost all patients experience improvements in their health parameters, and body-weight drops are more difficult to achieve. While some of my patients are certainly fast responders like Randi, others are very slow and even sometimes hardly responsive at all! The majority of my patients fall somewhere in between highly responsive and slower to respond.

From figure skating to disability

Melissa grew up being extremely athletic. She trained at a high level since she was very young and was serious about competitive figure skating. She regularly spent up to four hours daily skating throughout her childhood. And as she grew older she remained an avid athlete, running marathons and constantly working on fitness goals. In high school and college she was told by coaches that her body was "too big," that she weighed "too much," and she was advised to cut back her food and exercise even more. She saw her weight continue to climb and she was still on a diet when she first came to see me, weighing more than she ever had in her life. She watched everything she ate but her weight climbed to over 300 pounds. She was beyond frustrated and knew something was wrong.

We've worked together for years and have identified a big metabolism glitch most likely originating from the early diets, restrictive eating and excessive exercise since she was a little girl. Progress has been slow because medications are not powerful enough to reverse the problem significantly. Her medical complications include arthritis,

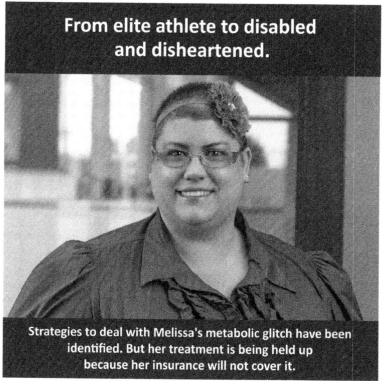

From elite athlete to disabled and disheartened.

Strategies to deal with Melissa's metabolic glitch have been identified. But her treatment is being held up because her insurance will not cover it.

asthma, sleep apnea and pulmonary blood clots. In Melissa's case her health problems and excess weight share a root cause—metabolic dysfunction. My hope is that we can combine medical and surgical treatment to correct her severe hormone imbalances. What are we waiting for? Her insurance won't cover it!

BACK TO NORMAL

As patients' metabolisms heal, their appetite, tastes, cravings, hunger-related sensations, and feelings of satisfaction normalize. One patient, Kay, shared with me, "I can't overstate how free I feel. Is this what normal people do? I feel like a normal human being for the first time. I can walk into the kitchen at work and candy doesn't call. I can get through the day. I don't feel deprivation around eating."

The body stops gaining weight when the metabolic signals make their way to the MC4Rs at Door Four of the metabolic pathway. And as the metabolism stabilizes, patients begin to lose weight automatically. When the metabolism normalizes, issues with blood pressure, cholesterol, or glucose usually improve significantly as well, even when no weight is lost.

MAKING PROGRESS AFTER 27 YEARS: CLAUDIA'S STORY

"Twenty-seven years ago I gained one hundred pounds in one year, even though I didn't change my diet or exercise," Claudia told me the first time we met. "I have been trying to figure out how to lose that weight ever since."

She tried various diets with no success, including one extreme diet, before deciding to go to one of the most prominent medical centers in the United States. Claudia was shocked and dismayed when the head of the center's

Division of Endocrinology, Diabetes, Metabolism, and Nutrition advised: "If you hire a personal trainer to work with you twice a week for forty-five minutes of isometric exercise and follow a 1,400 calorie diet, I have no doubt that you will lose four pounds per month." Claudia knew very well from experience that this advice wasn't going to solve her weight issues—she had tried even more extreme measures than this in the past, and none of them had worked.

When Claudia came to me, I initially saw metabolic problems, including Diet Fog, and soon after that I also discovered that she had leptin resistance. Gradually it became clear that she had an MC4R (Door Four) malfunction. It was also evident that, prior to her weight increase, she had been given a medication that disrupted a section of her metabolic pathway, which was probably what triggered her sudden weight gain. After all those years of failed diets, and after another year of treatment with me, Claudia has finally begun to make progress on weight loss and metabolic rebalancing through medical treatment—and without dieting. The strategies we've implemented are working slowly and steadily, and we hope to be able to navigate an effective treatment for the long term. A concern is that we still do not understand why her Door Four is not working better. My suspicion is that the medication that was the original trigger may have caused a permanent change in her metabolic pathway. We hope to continue to make steady progress.

CHAPTER 12

Steps to A Healthy Metabolism

IN MORE THAN twenty-five years of practice I've never had a single patient develop diabetes under my care—including those who were at high risk for developing diabetes—who already had pre-diabetes or insulin resistance when they first came to see me. While it's nice to celebrate weight loss, as a physician I'm most interested in what is going on with blood pressure, cholesterol, blood sugar, fatty liver disease, and other high risk medical conditions. My first priority is always health. What's on the inside is what is most important.

I have adopted a strategy for helping patients achieve better metabolic function that is certainly more rewarding than the strategy I employed when I first approached this problem twenty years ago with a "calories in, calories out" mindset. This process is straightforward: apply known science and available tools; obtain objective testing through lab work; collect an in-depth patient history; and talk with and listen to the patient. Then I can see what the landscape shows in terms of opportunity to adjust hormonal misalignments in both hormonal levels and their reception throughout the body. The goal is to reconnect and strengthen the communication feedback loop between my patient's brain and body to gain metabolic balance. Sometimes this involves adjusting exercise programs or backing off on exercise altogether for a while. Other times it may involve eating a more balanced diet, including all food groups, focusing on fueling rather than deprivation or restriction, eating meals and snacks more frequently, or going to bed earlier. In most cases, it includes finding the most appropriate medications to cast, splint, support, and close the gaps that fragment the metabolic feedback loop in order to restore communication throughout the loop.

When this individualized approach is successful, weight maintenance gradually becomes easier, weight reduction becomes possible, and appetite regulation eventually becomes easy and natural—and regardless of changes in body weight, health problems that were associated with the underlying metabolic issues nearly always improve. In addition, energy levels and overall quality of life usually improve.

It's important to understand that this process is not a cakewalk for a physician or a patient. It takes patience, careful monitoring, and juggling variables to support the body through nourishment, sleep, and consistent medical treatment. Weight problems related to metabolic dysfunction are most often a chronic medical condition, and treatment is a process. So treatment won't look like taking a course of antibiotics for a sinus infection. Rather, it will be an ongoing process of evaluation and treatment, requiring frequent monitoring and updating.

THE POWER OF TEAMWORK
Step 1: Identifying the Problem

There are usually two issues at play when treating a weight problem—the original metabolic problem and the secondary effects caused by prolonged dieting and/or excessive exercise. Although we cannot yet clinically test for every hormone involved in the metabolic feedback loop, an objective workup provides valuable information that reveals the chessboard, so to speak, on which we are playing—allowing us to see where kinks and gaps in the metabolic pathway are likely blocking hormonal signals from getting through to the brain and back. I, as the physician, am on one side of the chessboard, and the patient's cagey weight-defense system is on the other, trying to outsmart us. Once we have the necessary information, we then determine which moves we should make to treat the affected areas of the pathway, always aiming to be one step ahead of our opponent.

Step 2: Make the Body Feel Nutritionally Secure

Regardless of whether lab results suggest Diet Fog (low leptin, low insulin, and usually high ghrelin) or point to the original metabolic problem (which varies among patients, but usually results in the brain and body perceiving that fuel is scarce or fat mass is too low), you must first shut down the body's weight-defense system before you can make any progress at all.

When it comes to healing metabolic issues, nutritional eating and well-fueled exercise have many benefits, but it's important to shift our thinking about food and exercise from weight goals to *health* goals. We do have weight goals, but the thinking and behavior that support those goals should not be based on deprivation or control. We don't want to further exacerbate the problems of an already weak, fragmented metabolic feedback loop by making the body feel deprived. So, fueling consistently, fueling exercise well, and avoiding dietary rigidity are critical to making the body feel nutritionally secure.

Adequate sleep is also important, because metabolic hormone balancing primarily occurs when we are asleep. These health-based principles and recommendations are exactly the same as the ones I provide to patients who are trying to recover metabolically and physically from anorexia. The goal is to restore their metabolic function and balance their weight to a healthy range. Patients who tell me they struggle with binge eating, emotional eating, stress eating, compulsive overeating, or boredom eating think they are dealing with behavioral issues, but what they are really dealing with are biological symptoms. Although weight problems are certainly not psychological, stress can physiologically divert metabolic activity away from the appetite and metabolism receptors, which can contribute to glitches in the central metabolic pathway. When we realign the malfunctioning hormones, the biology is restored to normal, and the issues considered "bad behaviors" cease to be a problem.

Step 3: A New View on Fueling and Sleep:

Prioritize Eating

This is the most counterintuitive principal, and the one that my new patients are most surprised to hear–but prioritizing eating is key to successful treatment. If you're going to deactivate your weight-defense system, your body needs to know that it can trust you to feed it. So put self-nourishment at the top of your to-do list. Plan when and how you will nourish yourself, rather than planning when and howyou will not nourish yourself. Have conversations with yourself about eating rather than not eating. Your brain and body are listening. If you nourish yourself as you say you will, in time they will learn to trust you. This means eating breakfast within an hour of waking and then eating every few hours throughout the day to fuel your body. Alternate meals and snacks, and include all food groups. Don't go hungry.

Eat for Health

Rather than associating food with weight, your new nutritional goal is to not cut calories, stick to a plan, or eat (or not to eat) a certain kind of food. I realize this sounds crazy to most people who are used to being told that dieting is mandatory for weight-loss, and that it's very difficult for most people to transition from a life of dieting to a life without diets. Many patients I see are still dieting and have a diet mentality about food, even if they think they do not. I work with dieticians, and together we help patients understand what "not dieting" really means. Patients like Janet, Kayla and Randi all had to work hard to let go of their deprivation mindset, and it can be difficult, so having a support system is very beneficial. Your new goal is to nourish your brain and body with balanced meals and snacks so reliably throughout the day that they stop transmitting starvation signals. As the starvation signaling dies down, important changes will begin to take place: you will think more clearly, and your mood and energy will improve. With medical assistance, your metabolism will begin to repair and restore itself, and instead of Diet Fog, the Metabolic Storm, and weight gain, you will begin to experience the benefits of healthy fuel burning.

Change Your Mindset

All foods provide us with fuel. In that sense–and because you now understand that hormonal imbalances, not food, are what cause your weight problem–there are no good or bad foods. The minute you start being rigid and making rules, you will either gravitate to "off-limits" foods more than ever before or you'll activate your body's weight-defense system, causing your metabolism to shut down. In a recent study, subjects were given the same milkshake, but one group was told it was a "sensible" 140-calorie shake and the other group an "indulgent" 620 calorie shake. The group that was told it was an "indulgent shake" showed a bigger drop in the 'hunger hormone' Ghrelin than the "sensible shake" group. This demonstrates that just a **mindset** of deprivation can actually prevent ghrelin from dropping.

IDENTICAL MILKSHAKES

A. Crumb, "Mind over milkshakes: Mindsets, not just nutrients, determine ghrelin response," Health Psychology (July, 2011), 30(4):424-429

Fuel Yourself Consistently and Steadily

Eat three balanced meals every day, plus two to four snacks, so you never deprive your brain and body of fuel. This translates into eating every three hours or so. If you do not adequately fuel your brain, it will slow your metabolism to protect itself. This means you cannot afford to skip any meals. Yes, people with normal metabolisms may occasionally skip meals, but they can get away with it because their body doesn't fear starvation. Their weight defense system isn't ready to engage at any moment the way yours is. And don't forget to eat before exercise to provide your body with fuel, and immediately after exercise to restore your muscles' carbohydrate (glycogen) stores for your next workout.

Eat from All Three Macronutrient Groups at Each Meal

Everyone feels better if they eat from all food groups. Carbs are the brain and body's primary source of fuel, and fat and protein, in addition to having many other beneficial functions, help to regulate the pace of digestion. You need all of these macronutrients to be healthy and to offset the effects of your underlying hormonal malfunctions. Whenever possible, vary your sources of macronutrients while emphasizing foods that provide steady nutrition and support health. For example, three to five servings of whole grains daily is associated with reduced risk of diabetes, cardiovascular disease, and weight gain.[1]

---

1. E.Q. Ye, S.A. Chacko, et al., "Greater whole-grain intake is associated with lower risk of type 2 diabetes, cardiovascular disease, and weight gain," Journal of Nutriton (July 2012),142(7), doi: 10.3945/jn.111.155325: 1304-1313

Eat to Feel Good

Vegan, pescatarian, omnivore—all of these eating choices are fine, as long as they're driven by what makes you feel your best rather than by some diet fad or false belief that they will solve your weight problem.

Eat for Enjoyment

Eating for enjoyment is healthy. This is often a challenge for people who have lived a life of rigid dieting, control, and deprivation. People who take time to enjoy food as part of their culture appear to have healthier metabolisms than most Americans. For example, the French and Italians fall much lower than Americans do in obesity rankings. And the Spanish eat very late at night—a supposed no-no in this country—and yet their obesity levels are far below ours. Traditionally, these other cultures don't have many strict rules about eating. Eating supports their lifestyle—it doesn't control it. So, if you want some ice cream, have some and enjoy it.

Get Adequate Sleep

Sleep is critical for health, metabolism, and weight regulation. It provides recovery from the day's activities, and it reboots your entire system so your body is prepared for the demands of the next day. During sleep, the body regenerates muscle mass, builds bones and lean mass, and many important hormones that regulate metabolism are secreted throughout the night. Optimal sleep improves metabolism, energy, and mood.

The amount of sleep you get can affect your hormone levels, which can affect your metabolism and your body weight.

Sleep 4.5 5.0 5.5 6.0 6.5 7.0 7.5 8.0 8.5 9.0 hours

Ghrelin levels   Leptin levels

Taheri, et al 2004

The anti-metabolism hormone ghrelin is secreted primarily between midnight and 2 a.m., and the pro-metabolism hormone leptin is usually secreted between 2 and 4 a.m. Falling asleep well before these hormones secrete is optimal for healthy hormone balance. Your hormone secretion schedule may change based on when you eat breakfast and when you eat the last meal of your day, however. If you have a job that requires an early morning wake time, it's best to have breakfast early. This will encourage your hormone cycles to complete earlier in the night, before you wake up. When hormone cycles become disrupted or if sleep duration is under seven hours, the result is usually a higher ghrelin response and a lower leptin response. Basically, inadequate sleep can contribute to weight gain and weight loss resistance, especially in people with obesity and excess weight. Sleep apnea can disrupt the quality of sleep and increase stress hormones during the night, leading to elevated ghrelin levels and low leptin, which can jack up the appetite and crash metabolism, contributing to weight gain. Getting evaluated and treated for sleep apnea can be very beneficial.

Step 4: All the Rest

Medications & Supplements: Refrain from taking over-the-counter medications and supplements without checking their metabolic impact. Even vitamin C can affect your metabolism by lowering leptin levels, and niacin and glucosamine have been found to increase glucose levels. Supplements labeled as good for weight management or for leptin are frequently the opposite of what would be beneficial to metabolism, so don't fall for the marketing hype. Also, discuss prescription medication alternatives with your healthcare provider since many prescription medications have an impact on metabolism.

Stress: Excessive stress can affect metabolism negatively so it's a great idea to incorporate stress management techniques as part of your routine. Even warm baths, stretching, meditation, gentle yoga, tai-chi, reading, or listening to music can be stress relievers.

Obesogens: Scientists have found that many familiar products we're exposed to every day may affect our health because they contain potential disease and obesity promoting chemicals like BPA, Phthalates, and arsenic, which are often referred to as obesogens.

BpA and Phthalates are found in food and beverage can liners, plastic food packaging, synthetic carpeting and vinyl flooring, fragrances and certain cosmetics. Even a store receipt can contain BpA that can affect your blood levels. Check the bottom of plastic containers for the recycling symbol. Scientists suggest that numbers 2, 4 and 5 are associated the least potential health risk.

And, interestingly, the gluten-free craze may be increasing our arsenic exposure, since many gluten-free products are rice based and rice is often high in arsenic.

Scientists still don't know the best advice to give regarding exposure to these chemicals. There are even some studies suggesting that very low-level exposure may be even more detrimental than high-level exposure because at low levels, the body may mistake these chemicals for *our own* hormones, which have low concentration but high potency in our body. In fact, even the Endocrine Society, a conservative medical organization, is working on a position statement currently that suggests there is no safe level of exposure. But women planning to become pregnant may want to limit their exposure by avoiding certain cosmetics, fragrances and food packaging. And you can reduce your baby's exposure by avoiding synthetic carpeting and vinyl flooring in baby's bedroom.

Gestational Diabetes: Genetics combined with environmental triggers can amplify a genetic tendency from one generation to the next. For example, if you have a family history of diabetes or obesity or you or your mother had gestational diabetes, you personally have a much greater chance of developing diabetes and obesity. The screening test we use for gestational diabetes in the United States does not identify all the women who are actually experiencing gestational diabetes. Most of the rest of the world follows the World Health Organization recommendation for a more in-depth screening test. If the United States used that test, we'd identify some level of gestational diabetes in nearly 20% of pregnancies. But the lower dose, brief screening test we currently use only identifies approximately 4% of pregnancies as being associated with gestational diabetes. That's why many pregnant women and their developing babies aren't being identified and treated. And, if you're

Treating metabolic dysfunction successfully...

 Patient   **Provider**

	Patient	Provider
Nutrition and Exercise	• Eat regularly, every 3 hours • All food groups • Fuel all exercise • Avoid chemical food additives	• Do not prescribe diets or underfueled exercise • Give clear guidelines: determine if exercise should be reduced or restricted
Stress	• Reduce stress	• Provide education or referrals
Sleep	• Sleep 8 hours	• Evaluate for sleep apnea
Gestational Diabetes	• Get regular prenatal care • Eat all food groups every few hours • Aim for mild to moderate activity • Fuel all exercise	• Screen for gestational diabetes • Use longer screening test for patients with family history of diabetes or obesity • If medical treatment indicated, consider low-dose insulin
Environmental Obesogens	• Reduce exposure to BPA, secondhand smoke, food additives, pesticides, phthalates (fragrances, personal products, synthetic carpeting, etc.)	• Provide education
Medications	• Refrain from taking OTC meds and supplements without checking metabolic impact	• Choose alternative medications that are metabolically benign

METABOLIC FUNCTION

©2015 Emily Cooper, M.D.

...requires a patient–provider partnership.

  Laboratory   **Pharmacology**

Evaluate fasting-state metabolism

- Glucose
- HBA1C
- Insulin
- Lipids & particles
- Metabolic panel
- TSH, T3, T4
- Reproductive hormones
- Leptin
- ACTH, Cortisol, MSH
- NPY, Ghrelin

Increase anorexigen action

MSH   Insulin

Leptin   Incretins

POMC/CART

Amylin

Evaluate fed-state metabolism
Mixed meal glucose and insulin tolerance test

Rule out low blood sugar reaction after eating

Decrease orexigen action

Ghrelin (circulating)

AgRP/NPY   GABA

ß - Endorphin

 Normal Blood Sugar

 Weight Balanced

 Cardiovascular Health

 Fertility

born to a mother with gestational diabetes, your risk of obesity and type 2 diabetes is significantly increased, and the mother's risk of developing full blown type 2 diabetes in her lifetime is about 60%.

So if you are pregnant and have family risk factors for gestational diabetes, make an effort to undergo the more in-depth screening rather than the simple screening test. One other thing to note about gestational diabetes is that if medication is necessary, insulin in many ways is thought to be the best treatment for the baby. Oral medications have unknown effects on the developing baby and they cross the barrier from mother to baby. Insulin, on the other hand, does not cross this barrier. Thus, while oral medications can certainly work for *mom's* blood sugar regulation, in spite of the stigma associated with taking insulin, many scientists and clinicians believe that low-dose insulin treatment during pregnancy is the best option for the *baby* if medication is necessary during pregnancy.

HELPING YOUR CHILD HAVE A HEALTHIER METABOLISM

School districts have begun sending out letters and alerts to parents when a child's BMI is over a certain level. This can be really devastating to kids, as well as parents. Be aware of weight gains and losses, but BMI is not the most reliable measurement. With growth spurts, it's perfectly normal to gain 5–10 pounds before every inch that a child grows. It appears that they are gaining too much weight, but their bodies are just prepping for a normal growth spurt. So weight gain that's a little out of proportion but followed by a change in height is a sign of normal development.

Parents should avoid talking about diets, or bodies, or weight in the house, even if it's not about themselves or their kids. It can leave a lasting impression on children if they start to associate being thin with beauty and being fat with ugliness. Focusing on what's on the inside rather than the outside is so important for kids during puberty, as their bodies are changing.

But certain children are at risk for abnormal weight gain and obesity. If mom had gestational diabetes, both mom and baby are at a higher risk of developing obesity and diabetes as well. And studies suggest that fertility treatment, which is not uncommon, may be associated with a marked increase in risk of gestational diabetes and a risk of higher body weight in childhood. There are many other contributing factors, both genetic and environmental, contributing to childhood obesity.

Growth periods are typical times when children can be affected by abnormal weight gain. When metabolism is disrupted due to glitches, the child may increase in body weight but the following height acceleration just doesn't proceed proportionally. The most common time to see this imbalance in a weight-prone child is during puberty, particularly during ages 9-14 for girls and 11-16 for boys. Unfortunately, when children are affected prior to age 9 or 10, they stand out at school and are often teased.

Jennifer: Frustrated at 14

I received this letter from concerned parents about their fourteen-year-old daughter whose weight was rapidly increasing to a severe obesity range and continued to climb. They represent so many families who are frustrated and confused about why their child is experiencing rapid weight increases, in spite of healthy habits and targeted efforts, often guided by medical professionals.

Jennifer's mother wrote:

> "Our 14 year old daughter has been struggling with weight since around 9 years of age. We have tried multiple programs as well as many doctors. She did a full blood work up and things appear fine. My husband and I are just so frustrated and worried about our daughter's health. We began discussing this with her pediatrician years ago and were continually told that she 'would grow out of it.' It is affecting her health and mobility and we don't know what to do."

I really enjoyed meeting Jennifer and her parents. Jennifer was beyond frustrated by her situation. Although she did have lab work in the past, she never had an evaluation of her metabolic system. For example, there were no measurements of insulin levels or leptin, ACTH or MSH and no evaluation of her glucose and insulin balance after meals. Based on a comprehensive workup, we quickly pinpointed a primary problem with the balance between her glucose and insulin levels, particularly after meals. I explained to Jennifer that her weight problem was not her fault by any means and that no diet or exercise program would have corrected the problem. She had a follow-up visit with her physician soon after we had made the diagnosis and when her physician pointed an accusatory finger at her and said "what are you doing about your weight problem young lady?" she literally shouted at her "it's not my fault!" How could a 14-year old possibly have done anything to herself to cause this, and how could she possibly correct these problems on her own? Needless to say, that was the last time that Jennifer saw that physician.

Fortunately, her parents were persistent and now we are all thrilled that by correcting this problem medically and not dieting or exercising to try to lose weight Jennifer has been very successful. She rapidly and immediately began to shed the excess weight, so far over 50 pounds in the first nine months, and I expect her to reach a normal weight within another year. With proper diagnosis and treatment of her metabolic problem, Jennifer should have a healthy metabolic system that stays on track before she leaves home for college.

Most people think that they should cut back on food if their children have a weight problem, but that is not the right answer. Just as with adults, deprivation diets are not recommended. Instead, have healthy snacks around the house so when kids go to grab something, there's always something nutritious there. Children need nutrition and a balanced diet with three meals and snacks to fuel normal growth development. And researchers have shown again and again that children and adolescents who dieted are more likely to have obesity when they are adults.

For medical reasons, you often can't prevent your child from becoming overweight or obese. It's not their fault, and it's not yours.

CREATING A HEALTHY HOME FOR KIDS
- Avoid diet, body, and weight talk
- Eat meals together
- Regular bedtime, eight hours or more of sleep
- Have plenty of healthy foods available

- For small children, avoid vinyl flooring and synthetic carpeting in bedroom and play areas
- Get screened for insulin resistance, prediabetes, metabolic syndrome and fatty liver

CONCLUSION

Science Never Sleeps

WHEN WE CONSIDER HOW we as a society view weight problems, we are living in medieval times—which is why I'm so thrilled to bring you up to date on what scientists have discovered and what that means for people who are dealing with overweight and obesity. In this expanded second edition I've pushed the reader to challenge the status quo even more. When I first began to tell this story over a decade ago, I was met with enormous resistance. But with each year that passes and each new study that receives mention in the popular press and, especially, with your voices sharing your own stories with friends, family, and co-workers, the idea that diets fail the majority of people is becoming less controversial in our society. A day will come when everyone knows it and then what will the diet industry do? Will insurers pay for medical treatment? Will medical students learn the facts and will patients routinely receive the care they need?

We now know that metabolism is regulated by a complex feedback loop with the brain as the CEO and the hormones as the messengers, and we have learned that glitches can occur along this feedback loop, impairing metabolism, promoting fat storage, and often causing the appetite to increase—the Metabolic Storm. We also know that there are strong genetic influences that increase weight-prone tendencies, and that in genetically vulnerable people glitches can be triggered by environmental factors, such as dieting (especially in childhood), sleep deprivation, certain medications, and endocrine-disrupting obesogens. These glitches are not within a person's control—they are a medical problem, and should be treated as such.

For nearly one hundred years, scientists have proven that diets don't "cure" overweight and obesity—and, worse, that they actually aggravate the problem by slowing metabolism and leaving a lasting fingerprint that encourages weight regain. According to multiple studies, even exercise cannot prevent this slowdown.

Healthcare providers, trainers, friends, family, and co-workers who recommend diets are well-meaning—but they often fail to realize that while dieting may seem to work in the short term, long-term maintenance of weight lost through dieting is generally unrealistic.

It has been nearly a century since physicians and scientists first began to explore the metabolic causes and potential treatments of obesity. We have finally discovered and isolated numerous hormone messengers and brain components involved in metabolism and proven their actions and interactions, uncovering the peripheral and central metabolic pathways. We now have treatments available to realign the metabolic feedback loop, with promising advances on the horizon. Science is catching up to the impressive insight of those endocrinologists of the 1920s who challenged the thinking of their time—and we are now making real progress in this area of medicine.

What we have learned from studying weight problems and metabolism is that the perceptions many of us have of people confronted with overweight and obesity are often *mis*perceptions. Weight and health are not necessarily related: you can be healthy or fit at any weight, and unhealthy or unfit at any weight. And while it's nice to celebrate weight loss, it's what's on the inside that is most important.

The brain of a person with obesity is essentially blind to the excess weight the body is carrying, and this can lead to preoccupation with food and impaired satisfaction after eating. So, like the excess weight itself, increased appetite is a symptom of an underlying problem. That's why simply dieting or using discipline to control food intake does not fix the problem long term.

Medical conditions are associated with specific symptoms and abnormal test findings, and are addressed with medical treatment. Based on that definition, obesity is a medical condition. If the thyroid is not functioning normally, we take thyroid hormones to stay in optimal ranges. If we have an infection, we use antibiotics to eradicate it. If we have a tumor, we perform surgery or chemotherapy to reduce its size. So when it comes to overweight and obesity, why don't we apply the same perspective?

Given the fact that we're facing an epidemic of diabesity, it's imperative that we act to prevent it. Today science offers so much hope for people experiencing weight problems. Over the next decade scientists will be busy refining more synthetic hormones and agents that block or accentuate hormone action, and will be coming up with other strategies that retrain and normalize metabolic function.

The more we know about how the metabolism works, the more obvious it is that weight problems are medical problems and they are not anyone's fault. Most patients could already benefit from treatments that exist today—but there is still progress to be made.

Thankfully for us, science never sleeps.

End Notes

Chapter 5 Timeline Sources:

KS Polonsky, "The Past 200 Years in Diabetes," New England Journal of Medicine (2012) Vol. 367 No. 14: 1332–1340 doi:10.1056/NEJMra1110560, PDF on file.

D.V. Fenby, "Heat: Its measurement from Galileo to Lavoisier," *Pure and Applied Chemistry* (1987), Vol. 59, No.1: 91—100.

G Eknoyan, "Adolphe Quetelet (1796–1874)—The Average Man and Indices of Obesity," Nephrolpgy Dialysis Transplantation (2008) Vol. 23: 47–51. doi:10.1093/ndt/ gfm517, PDF on file.

E.A.M Gale, "Timeline 1900-1950," Diapedia (July 27, 2013), 1104709121 Rev. No. 7.

A. Mazur, "Why were 'starvation diets' promoted for diabetes in the pre-insulin period?," Nutrition Journal (2011), 10:23, doi: 10.1186/1475-2891-10-23.

LH Peters. Diet and Health With Key to the Calories. 1918 The Reilly & Britton Co. (USA)

B.W. McGuinness, "Melanocyte-Stimulating Hormone: A Clinical And Laboratory Study," Annals of the New York Academy of Sciences (December 15, 2006), DOI: 10.1111/j.1749-6632.1963.tb42921.x.

Nobelprize.org, The Discovery of Insulin, http://www. nobel prize.org/educational/medicine/insulin/discovery-insulin .html.

IW Campbell, "Metformin-life Begins at 50. Symposium of 43rd Meeting European Association for the Study of Diabetes," The British Journal of Diabetes and Vascular Disease (2007) Vol. 7: 247-252   PDF on file.

N.R. Gosmanov, A.R. Gosmanov, J.E. Gerich, Glucagon Physiology, Endotext.org (February 4, 2011), http://www .endotext.org/diabetes/diabetes2/diabetes2.html.

H. Lisser, "The Frequency Of Endogenous Endocrine Obesity And Its Treatment By Glandular Therapy," *California and Western Medicine* (October 1924), Vol. XXII, No. 10: 509-514.

M. Sattley, "The History of Diabetes," *Diabetes Health* (November 1996).

DK Burnham, "Insulin and Insulin Mixtures—NPH Insulin," California Medicine 1951 (1951) Vol. 75 No. 6: 412-415

V. C. Medvei, "Chronological Tables," *History of Clinical Endocrinology* (Taylor & Francis, January 1, 1993), 488.

S.S. Londhe, "A Major Health Hazard: Metabolic Syndrome," *International Journal of Pharmacy and Pharmaceutical Sciences* (2011), ISSN-0975-1491, Vol. 3, Issue 3: 1-8.

Thebariatricsurgeryresource.com, *The History of Bariatric Surgery,* http://thebariatricsurgeryresource.com/articles/2012/03/06/history-bariatric-surgery.

IW Campbell, "Metformin-life Begins at 50. Symposium of 43rd Meeting European Association for the Study of Diabetes," The British Journal of Diabetes and Vascular Disease (2007) Vol. 7: 247-252

"Science: Simulated ACTH," *Time,* December 12, 1960.

Recent Prog Horm Res. 1973;29:457-96. Endocrine and metabolic effects of experimental obesity in man. Sims EA, Danforth E Jr, Horton ES, Bray GA, Glennon JA, Salans LB. PMID: 4750591

B.A. Ramlo-Halsted, S.V. Edelman, "The Natural History of Type 2 Diabetes: Practical Points to Consider in Developing Prevention and Treatment Strategies," *Clinical Diabetes* (2000), Vol. 18 No. 2: 80-84.

K. Tatemoto, "Neuropeptide Y: History and Overview", ed. M.C. Michel, *Neuropeptide Y and Related Peptides* (Springer, 2004): 2-12.

S. Zac-Varghese, T. Tan, S. R. Bloom, "Hormonal Interactions Between Gut and Brain," *Discovery Medicine* (Dec 26, 2010).

T. J. Kieffer, J. F. Habener, "The Glucagon-Like Peptides," *Endocrine Reviews* (December 1, 1999), doi: 10.1210/ er.20 .6.876, Vol. 20 No. 6: 876-913.

G.J. Cooper, A.C. Willis, A. Clark, et al., "Purification and characterization of a peptide from amyloid-rich pancreases of type 2 diabetic patients," Proceedings of the National

Academy of Sciences of the United States of America (December 1987), PMCID: PMC299599: 8628–8632.

US Neill, "Leaping for leptin: the 2010 Albert Lasker Basic Medical Research Award goes to Douglas Coleman and Jeffrey M. Friedman," Journal of Clinical Investigation (2010) Vol. 120 No. 10: 3413-3418

Medicalnews.net, Metformin, http://www.news-medical.net/health/Metformin-History.aspx.

JJ Diez and P Iglesias, "The Role of the Novel Adipocyte-derived Hormone Adiponectin in Human Disease," European Journal of Endocrinology (2003) Vol. 148: 293-300

Solomon Sobel, Director—Center For Drug Evaluation and Research, to Jennifer Stotka, Director, U.S. Regulatory Affairs—Eli Lilly and Company, September 11, 1998.

J.B. Hillman, J. Tong, M. Tschop, "Ghrelin Biology and Its Role in Weight-related Disorders," Discovery Medicine (June 17, 2011).

R. A. Pittner, A. A. Young, J. R. Paterniti, Jr., "Methods of treating obesity using PYY," U.S. Patent Application (December 14, 2001).

S.R. Bloom, et al., "Oxyntomodulin for preventing or treating excess weight," U.S. Patent Application (September 9, 2002).

M. Nauck, "Type 2 Diabetes: Principles and Practice, Second Edition," eds. B.J. Goldstein, D. Mueller-Wieland, *Type 2 Diabetes,* (CRC Press, November 14, 2007): 159.

T.E. Gottschalk Boeving, S. Klysner, "Immunization against autologous ghrelin," U.S. Patent Application (September 12, 2003).

"New GLP-1 analogs, mimetics in the pipeline for type 2 diabetes," *Endocrine Today,* May 2009.

M.C. Jones, "Therapies for Diabetes: Pramlintide and Exenatide," *American Family Physician* (June 15, 2007), 75(12): 1831-1836.

Bms.com, "U.S. FDA Grants Priority Review to Bristol-Myers Squibb and AstraZeneca's Metreleptin, an Investigational Agent for Treatment of Metabolic Disorders Associated with Rare Forms of Lipodystrophy," http://news.bms.com/press-release/us-fda-grants-priority-review-bristol-myers-squibb-and-astrazenecas-metreleptin-invest.

Chapter 9 References:

Chandra A, Copen CE, Stephen EH. Infertility and impaired fecundity in the United States, 1982–2010: Data from the National Survey of Family Growth. National health statistics reports; no 67. Hyattsville, MD: National Center for Health Statistics. 2013

Travison TG, AB Araujo, AB O'Donnell, et al., "A Population-level Decline in Serum Testosterone Levels in American Men," Journal of Clinical Endocrinology and Metabolism (2007), Vol. 92 No. 1: 196-202, doi: 10.1210/jc.2006-1375

Michalakis K, G Mintziori, A Kaprara, et al., "The Complex Interaction Between Obesity, Metabolic Syndrome and Reproductive Axis: A Narrative Review," Metabolism (2013), Vol. 62 No. 4: 457-478

Messini CI, K Dafopoulos, M Malandri, et al., "Inhibioty Effect of Submaximal Doses of Ghrelin on Gonadotropin Secretion in Women," Hormone and Metabolic Research (2014), Vol. 46 No. 1: 36-40, doi: 10.1055/s-0033-1355388

Greenman Y, Rouach V, Limor R, et al. Testosterone is a strong correlate of ghrelin levels in men and postmenopausal women. Neuroendocrinology. (2009) Vol 89 No. 1:79-85. doi: 10.1159/000151768. Epub 2008 Aug 28.

Hausman GJ, Barb CR, Lents CA. Leptin and reproductive function. Biochimie. (2012) Vol 94:2075-2081

Patarrão RS, Lautt WW, Macedo MP. Assessment of methods and indexes of insulin sensitivity. Rev Port Endocrinol Diabetes Metab. 2014;9(1):65–73

Chen M, Norman RJ, Heilbronn LK. Does in vitro fertilisation increase type 2 diabetes and cardiovascular risk? Curr Diabetes Rev. (2011) Vol 7 No. 6:426-432

Ashrafi M, R Gosili, R Hosseini, et al., "Risk of Gestatonal Diabetes Mellitus in Patients Undergoing AssistedRepro- ductive Techniques," European Journal of Obstetrics & Gynecology and Reproductive Biology (2014), Vol. 176: 149-152

Nijher GK, WS Dhillo, SR Bloom. "Kisspeptin: A Novel Role in the Regulation of Reproductive Function," Drug News Perspective (2009), Vol. 22 No. 10: 573-578, doi:10.1358/ dnp.2009.22.10.1434630

Stevens A, G Begum, A White, "Epigenetic Changes in the Hypothalamic Pro-opiomelanocortin Gene: A Mechanism Linking Maternal Undernutrition to Obesity in the Offspring?" European Journal of Pharmacology (2011), Vol. 660 No. 1: 194-201, doi: 10.1016/j.ejphar.2010.10.111

ACKNOWLEDGMENTS

I COULD NOT HAVE WRITTEN this book without the passion, trust, and commitment of all my patients. In the early years of my clinical practice at Seattle Performance Medicine hundreds of patients faithfully tracked their food intake, hunger levels, exercise, and sleep. Together, we discovered that diets simply don't work long term, and we searched for other, more successful, treatments. Some patients' problems were particularly difficult to diagnose, but we persistently worked together to find and target underlying metabolic glitches. Thanks to these earlier patients who never gave up, many others have benefited from what we learned along the pathway of discovery.

It takes great courage, curiosity, and determination to have faith in a new process. But my patients never stopped believing that, through science, we could diagnose and treat their underlying metabolic problems. And by understanding how their metabolism operated, they were finally freed from deprivation dieting forever.

I am grateful to those courageous patients who are willing to share their personal stories so that readers with similar issues might know that they are not alone and that help is possible. I am especially grateful to Bea, who convinced me—twenty years ago—that the body is capable of healing itself. Bea suffered from obesity and nearly lost her life several times due to complications from past treatment. She inspired me to believe in the body's healing capabilities and never to underestimate its power to survive—and even thrive—in spite of extraordinarily adverse circumstances.

Thank you, Dr. Hans Lisser and the other 20th-century pioneers in the field of metabolism and obesity, for challenging popular assumptions with real science and inspiring me to continue my search for new, science-based solutions to our Diabesity Epidemic. And thank you, present-day experts, my colleagues, and my mentors. I value the insight, and support you generously provide.

My family has always encouraged me to follow my dreams and be a brave explorer, even if my pursuits might lead to facts that challenge the status quo. Thanks to them for their unconditional love and their assurance that everything is possible, and for urging me to always seek the truth and act upon it, regardless of popular opinion.

Thank you to my talented team—Andrea Taylor, Beret Hamilton, and Jan Cooper— whose tenacity, creativity, and focus brought this book to life. And to my illustrator, Dory Rikkonen, whose brilliance is self-explanatory, and Janet Frohnmayer and Debra Cotter, who helped organize drafts of the book. I also thank Brooke Warner and Tabitha Lahr for their expert assistance. I couldn't have accomplished so much without you all.

Finally, I am indebted to Joyce Taylor, Emmy-award-winning anchor, for her insight and compassion toward those affected with obesity and infertility. She has provided a media platform where our non-profit Foundation can share the exciting science of metabolism with the Seattle community and beyond.

ABOUT THE AUTHOR

DR. EMILY COOPER, Seattle-based physician with more than twenty years of experience, is board-certified in three specialties: Family Medicine, Sports Medicine, and Obesity Medicine. Dr. Cooper developed her clinical skills during medical school at London Hospital Medical College in England. There, she learned to combine an investigative approach with scientific analysis to obtain a comprehensive view of each of her patients.

In the late 1980s, while completing her residency at a community hospital in Pennsylvania, Dr. Cooper became interested in emerging research that associated several health conditions with increased body weight. She was excited to learn that metabolic imbalances such as metabolic syndrome and insulin resistance were the root cause of many health concerns and were most likely reversible and preventable. This opened up a new avenue for making a difference in preventing obesity, diabetes, heart attacks, and strokes.

Dr. Cooper's interest in metabolism and obesity grew in the 1990s, when she realized that some of her patients gained weight while making efforts to lose, or at the very least, maintain their weight. Looking back, she says it was an oversimplification to think that all she needed to do to help her patients lose weight was to educate them about healthy eating and exercise. In spite of her efforts to perfect the "calories in, calories out" formula, individualizing it for each patient, Dr. Cooper found that regardless of how much weight a patient lost, it always came back.

Dr. Cooper's persistence over the past twenty years has led her to challenge antiquated assumptions and embrace a scientific perspective with the goal of more effectively treating metabolic causes of obesity, diabetes and infertility. Today, most of her patients have experienced significant improvements as a result of applying a scientific approach instead of engaging in dieting and exercise weight-loss strategies.

In the course of her work with patients and their families, Dr. Cooper formed the new Cooper Center for Metabolism, a division of Seattle Performance Medicine, specializing in treatment of the metabolic causes of obesity, diabetes, and infertility.

She is convinced that the evidence in support of a science-based approach to obesity and metabolic malfunction needs a stronger voice to gain the attention of the healthcare community, the media, and the general public. Therefore, in an effort to provide a sounding board for the science of metabolism and its importance in reversing the country's Diabesity Epidemic, Dr. Cooper founded The Diabesity Research Foundation, a 501c3 non-profit organization focused on publishing scientific case reports and educating healthcare providers and the public on Diabesity and its diagnosis and treatment. Health experts predict that the Diabesity Epidemic—a public health crisis characterized by the combined epidemics of obesity and type 2 diabetes—will affect up to 60 percent of the U.S. adult population by 2020. Changing this trajectory starts with education and depends on open conversation among friends, family members, patients and their doctors, and scientists and the community.

In Dr. Cooper's view, it is only by basing prevention and treatment on the underlying causes of obesity that we can achieve meaningful overall health. Dr. Cooper hopes that with a greater public awareness of the science of metabolism and obesity, we will move away from antiquated assumptions and ineffective, potentially harmful treatments and redirect our efforts towards the findings of pure science.

CPSIA information can be obtained
at www.ICGtesting.com
Printed in the USA
LVOW13s0251260117

522226LV00030B/577/P

9 780989 690201